The  BodyJoy Plan

The 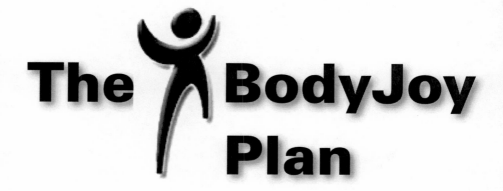 BodyJoy Plan

Your Solution to Fat Loss, Health & Happiness

Mindy P. Buxton, CSCS

To order additional copies of this book, contact:
Xlibris Corporation
1-888-795-4274
www.Xlibris.com
Orders@Xlibris.com
63675

Table of Contents

MIND

MOVEMENT

MEALS

Book Testimonials

"I like the overall approach of this book. It is psychologically sound and it's very cognitively based. It also addresses a number of psychological barriers which are important for seeing successful changes."

—Jeff Sheffield, Psychologist

"In the words of a popular TV personality, Mindy's 'get real' approach to health and fitness is refreshing! Having 'walked the walk' herself, Mindy has a unique ability to take you by the hand and help you with your fitness goals. It's rare (especially in book form) to feel like a true friend is there to guide you along—no matter where you're starting from. 'Overcoming Bad Body Days' (Strategy 4) was a real breakthrough for me personally, and I've been going to the gym for most of my adult life! You'll find this entire book talking about you for a change!"

—Preston Christensen, Successful Business Owner & Retired Athlete

"I lost 18.5 inches, 11 pounds and 3 percent body fat by following Mindy's 6-week plan. This book has changed my life!"

—Nanette Westley, Elementary School Teacher

Client Testimonials

"I have trained with Mindy for four years and have not only lost a lot of weight and inches, I have enjoyed the workouts. She keeps me focused (even though she knows I love my wine). I feel and look like a new person."

—Holly Elliot, 53, Realtor

"Mindy is fun and filled with energy, which filters out to those around her. She makes me work out hard and safely."

—Sheridan Shiffigen, 20, Student

"Through my experience with training, I have really enjoyed the commitment that comes along with training. I have enjoyed the opportunity to go to the gym twice a week without fail. Mindy's constant uplifting attitude was always a wonderful help and always pushed me that extra bit to get in shape. She always had encouraging comments that made me want to do better. The workouts she had me do always focused on areas I needed improvement in. I really enjoyed each workout and exercise was made enjoyable and fun. She is a great support to me as my husband is going through cancer treatment. She reminds me of how important managing stress is and how much keeping myself fit and healthy will help me through this time."

—Carla Jenkins, 54, Mom, Grandma, and Florist

"My favorite belief I have learned from Mindy is that fitness isn't about a number on the scale or what size you are. She has taught me that it is about being healthy. It's how, what and the portion sizes you eat. It's positive thinking in everyday life; what you tell yourself; how you perceive the world. It's getting in your cardio as well as your weights, and being committed to doing those things daily. Through her example she has shown me how to have a sound body and mind so that I can accomplish anything I choose. Mindy and I have been doing the unthinkable (in my mind). We have been training for a marathon, something I never thought I'd do. I can honestly say it has been an awesome experience—one I couldn't have done without her support. Running with a partner is inspiring. Mindy has helped me continuously put effort into my goal. My self-esteem has shot through the roof knowing I've accomplished my goal. I have become a better person by knowing Mindy, and I've been blessed to have her help as my trainer and running partner. I thank her for that! I hope I can be the kind of influence to those around me that Mindy has been to me."

—Jen Dyer, 27, Mother of four

"I have battled my weight my whole life. I was very intimidated to join a gym. When I did, I met Mindy. When I first met her she was expecting her second child—I couldn't believe what great shape she was in! Her positive attitude inspired me to try spinning classes. I never thought I could take a spin class and survive! Mindy was so patient with me. She helped me start slow and learn to pace myself. Mindy's class is now my favorite and I've consistently lost weight since I started spinning with her. I am so thankful for the opportunity to work out with such a positive person. I always feel wonderful at the end of class. Thank you, Mindy, for inspiring me to work out and, more importantly, believe in myself."

—Chrisanne Sueltz, 37, Business Owner

"It's not hard for me to express my positive opinion of my time training with Mindy. From the beginning she evaluated my goals and expectations of my desired results with training. She knew and carefully evaluated all of my physical limitations, never causing undo pain, soreness or injury. Yet, she pushed me hard enough to where I could see and feel results. I always felt she kept up-to-date on realistic food choices and healthy everyday, realistic nutrition choices. She is always up beat, happy and I always feel better physically and mentally when I am done with my training session. I also feel confident in her knowledge of exercises, anatomy, and the proper way to achieve results in improving the weight and muscle tone of my body. I would recommend her to anyone with the highest degree of confidence."

—Brenda Morris, 55, Mother and Grandmother

"I have always appreciated Mindy's professional and supportive attitude with my training. Her very pleasant approach to training actually motivates me and helps me look forward to our training sessions. I appreciate that Mindy 'does her homework' on new trends in personal training. She is always suggesting helpful new things to do."

—Dr. Leon Hansen, 51, OB/GYN

"I am a former professional volleyball player and I moved from Italy to Utah in 1999 with my husband (a retired professional basketball player). I met Mindy at the LifeCentre Athletic Club, just after she had her first baby. I remember thinking how persistent and dedicated she was not only with her clients but with herself. I remember noticing how fast she was able to get back into shape and how her clients were making amazing improvements. I know most of Mindy's clients and they have gone through some incredible changes these past years, not only with their bodies, but their attitudes and confidence levels as well. I've had the luck to train with Mindy as a workout partner and even though I've lifted weights for many years and have also played competitive athletics, she definitely finds good ways to challenge me. She has shown me many new exercises and training techniques that have made my workouts challenging and fun. What really makes Mindy a great trainer is her willingness to continually improve herself and learn about everything new out there in her field. She is knowledgeable, competent, and she has taught me much both as a trainer and as a friend. My husband and I have come to know Mindy very well these past few years and we have much respect and admiration for what she does as a trainer, and we also love her for who she is. She's an amazing trainer and precious friend."

—Gaia and Pace Mannion,
former Professional Volleyball and NBA player

9/2/04

"Dear Mindy:

Many thanks for your knowledge, patience, and perseverance these past six years. You always told me I should work on the following items in order to be successful. You said:

- *Watch your stress level*
- *Stay motivated*
- *Follow sound nutritional guidelines*
- *Exercise regularly*
- *Get the proper amount of sleep*
- *Drink plenty of water*

I have done some of the things above at one time or another and I have met successes and failures. A summer ago, I was told I should have a knee replacement by spring, I finally decided to work on all of the items listed above and I have found great success. It hasn't even been hard either! By making small changes along the way, I have been able to continuously improve. I have focused on what to do rather than those things I should've been doing. I found that eating enough fiber in my fruits and vegetables really kept me from being hungry. The water helped me feel full and function better also.

I have tried to reduce my stress level—exercising regularly has been good for this as well as many other things. I have toned up my muscles and have lost inches, weight, and fat percent. I'm back into my smallest size clothes.

Having enough sleep has kept my energy level up during the day and kept me sharper.

All I know is that by following your plan my life has become much better. (I have even been able to put off that knee surgery for now!) Thank you again, Mindy! You've done so much for me!

With much love and admiration,

Nanette Westley

Your client and former 4th grade teacher

Age 64"

Dedicated to

My husband, TJ Buxton, who constantly inspires me to do the impossible.

My girls, Alexis and Elle Buxton for making my life complete.

My entire family for their unconditional support.

My training clients, whom I care for as much as my family.

And all other individuals who seek to be happy, fit and healthy in their best body.

Acknowledgements

Thank you's are in order to a number of people who have supported me and contributed to this book. First and foremost, TJ Buxton: Thanks for giving me the encouragement to do something I never thought I could. Thank you for sacrificing your time and for being so supportive. You make me a better person and I'm glad I have you as my best friend, spouse, colleague, and support system. Thanks for helping me be my best and for making me so happy.

Thank you mom and dad for your never-ending support, love and encouragement. I appreciate all you do for me and my girls.

A special thank you to Vicki Linton, my nutrition advisor and faithful client. I am grateful for all the advice, knowledge and time you spent assisting me on this as well as all other "projects" I dream up. You are a wonderful person and I enjoy watching you accomplish your dreams and goals.

Thanks to Mark Green, business partner and friend. Thanks for helping me find clarification and direction when I need it most. I benefit greatly from your "tough love" and honesty—sometimes brutal, but always necessary. Thanks for your time, ideas and friendship. Everyone needs a Greener!

Thanks to my BodyGym family. To Doug, for providing me with opportunities and sparking ideas that weren't there before. For the inspiration I received from the BodyGym Challenges. To the participants who gave me hope and happiness watching their success. For the results I've had with my BodyGym. I am a better person and trainer for the journey I have been on with you.

A much deserved thank you to Melanie, Jeff, Carol, Nan, Preston, and the many others who have spent time editing, contributing, and assisting me with this book to make it a useful tool for those who are interested in improving their bodies and lives.

Thank you to my clients. You are inspiring and have helped me so much over the years. Thanks for your hard work, dedication, commitment and the time you spend reaching your goals. I appreciate the friendships and growth I have received from knowing you.

Last, but not least, thanks to my personal trainer, John. Thank you for showing me what a difference one person can make in the lives of others. Thanks for the support and friendship you show me and for the example you are. Thanks for helping me find my way to the most satisfying and rewarding job there is outside of my family.

Introduction

When I started gathering my thoughts for this book, a friend read a quote to me that stayed in my mind throughout the writing process: "People don't need another diet book, or piece of equipment, they need a new experience." Isn't that the truth! This book was created out of the frustration that I didn't have a single, solid resource for my training clients to find healthy ways to improve their figure, and meet their goals. They were reading all the fad books, but kept experiencing yo-yo dieting. An abundance of diet information is out there, but nothing that helped create healthy, long-term results, and a joyful experience.

As I reflected on my own journey to BodyJoy, I discovered that the information I was sharing with others was not the typical diet information, or rigid instructions on what to do for a workout and what to eat; it was strategies that helped them create *new experiences* in order to build their best bodies. This is information that can work for anyone. You don't need to waste time or money searching for the answers. The answers for your success are inside of you, and I will help you bring those answers to a place where you can work with them, and create success, joy, and greater health that will last a lifetime.

Needless to say, this book is not about dieting: *it's about you*. I created it to provide you with doable, realistic strategies that can help you find happiness, accomplishment and satisfaction, by finding your best body. This book will create your new experience of succeeding and overcoming dieting.

We often deal with struggle, restraint, dissatisfaction, and punishment associated with our bodies and food. I want to provide you with the right strategies so you can experience satisfaction, fulfillment and freedom with your body, and your relationship with food. It's time to experience BodyJoy! In these pages you will find information that is doable—no matter who you are or what your situation is. This time you will experience long-term change and improvements!

Although marketing approaches make success look simple and instant, I understand how the struggle to achieve your best body can seem never-ending. I know because I've been there. I know how frustrating it is to work on changing your body for a long period of time and see no results. I know what it feels like to be unhappy and unhealthy.

I've watched hundreds of training clients take on the challenge to achieve their best body and work on goals to help them look, feel and function better. To lose body fat and inches is a challenge. It does take effort. However, the challenge doesn't have to be as unpleasant as "dieting." You will be surprised at how small, basic changes will lead to drastic results!

Based on the hundreds of clients I've trained, and on the fact you are reading this book, it's safe to say you are striving for two things: to *look* better and to *feel* better. These aspirations sound simple, yet due to past dieting experiences and all the distractions and fad tips that are available, achieving them can be difficult.

My plan will deliver your best body. It won't happen overnight. Contrary to the promises of most quick-fix plans, it will take longer than a few days or a week. However, this time you will receive a great benefit—the opportunity to create your best body and the knowledge, skills, and tools to maintain it for the rest of your life. Long-term results that will make you look and feel better, and function at your best!

This is The BodyJoy Plan.

Unlike other plans, BodyJoy is based on simplicity. Incorporating my three essential elements to losing inches and body fat: **Mind, Movement, and Meals**.

These three basic concepts are key—and the way they are understood and implemented makes all the difference in the world. When you create balance with all three, you will be able to achieve long-term fat-loss and experience BodyJoy.

When it comes to long-term results, the will to achieve is important, but the will to prepare is *vital.*

Preparation though, doesn't have to be difficult or time consuming. BodyJoy offers a simple, realistic approach towards meeting your physical goals—no matter who you are or what you do. Welcome to The BodyJoy Plan.

Are You Really Ready—To Make a Change?

Permanent fat loss and finding your best body requires small but important modifications to the way you live your life. Are you ready to make these modifications? Are you ready this very moment to ignore "quick-fix" dieting and fad diet plans? Are you ready to understand which type of eater you are and take necessary action to change that behavior? Are you ready to change your thinking regarding food and its purpose and/ or meaning in your life? Are you ready to learn how to set and achieve realistic goals?

Are you willing to learn how to be happy regardless of your size? Are you ready to control your environment (kitchen, house, or desk) and not let your environment control you? Are you willing to learn how simple preparation leads to long-term results? Are you willing to make activity part of your regular, daily schedule? Are you willing to adopt a positive attitude towards exercise and admit that fitness is something you will need to work on for the rest of your life? Are you ready to improve your quality of life? Are you ready to start *RIGHT NOW*? Great! Let's begin.

Mind

Mental and emotional elements must be in place before you can succeed in your health and fat-loss goals. A healthy mind leads to a healthy body. Many body issues, such as gaining weight, not liking yourself, or feeling unfulfilled are not directly related to food; they are related to how you think and deal with emotions, self-respect, fears, problems and stress. Many of the obstacles you face when trying to improve your body stems from mental stumbling blocks, not physical ones. Almost daily you can hear or read, "Eat healthy foods and exercise regularly." This is common knowledge. You know you need to do it, but you haven't yet discovered *how* to actually do it. BodyJoy teaches you *how*.

"Success must be felt on the inside before it can be seen on the outside."

—Anonymous

Through personal training and life coaching I've learned that seeing results are not just a matter of what people eat or how much they exercise. Not only do I counsel my clients on nutrition, exercise, and fitness, but I get to help them see the "big picture" of their lives and help them repair any pieces that may be broken or out of balance. These are usually the reasons why they diet and can't reach their goals long-term. Wellness or well-being plays a large part in achieving long-term success and happiness. These elements are directly affected by our minds in our thoughts and beliefs. Much of our success depends on our mindset.

The choices you make each day have a powerful effect on your health and well-being. What you eat, your level of exercise and movement, and how you manage stress, are just a few of the choices you face daily.

By changing or refocusing your mind or your perception, you can change anything in your life, including your size. This allows you to take control. You can make your body into what you would like it to be, as opposed to feeling as if your body is in control of you. These changes do not need to be all or nothing. They don't have to take place all at once. By simply changing a few food habits, or by walking a few more steps than usual, you can improve your figure and overall health. Do what you are capable of now and know that when you are ready, you will implement more changes in the future. The important thing is that you begin.

Understand that your current nutrition and exercise habits are behavioral (you have learned them). They are affected by what you do or don't do on a regular basis. Becoming leaner, healthier and experiencing more happiness comes from making small changes. These results do not come from extreme dieting or restrictions.

BodyJoy Tip

Within you right now is the power to do things you never dreamed possible. This power becomes available to you just as you can change your beliefs."

- Maxwell Maltz

BodyJoy provides you with several, realistic strategies you will implement into your life at your own pace. Of course, the more strategies you implement, the faster you will see results. Don't be overwhelmed by thinking you have to learn an entire new way of eating or exercising. You'll be surprised at how simple it is to start seeing results. Remember, basic improvements you make in your behavior or lifestyle will give you a better life experience and your best body.

Let the strategies begin!

Strategy 1

The BodyJoy Mindset: Leaving the
"Weight-Loss Mentality" Behind

Let's take on your first change together: weight loss. However, weight loss will not be the main focus in achieving your results. This is a secret to success!

The most important change you will make is to transfer your attention *away* from weight loss and *on* to wellness. Leave your weight loss mindset behind. In wellness, we assess body composition. Body composition is more than the number of pounds you weigh: it refers to the relative proportions by weight of your body's fat mass compared to its lean, or fat-free, mass. The healthiest way to assess your body composition is through testing your body fat percentage or by using the waist to hip ratio. See my website for details on testing body composition, *www.mindybuxton.com.*

Expect to see inch loss, expect to go down in clothing sizes, and expect to lose body fat. These changes will be permanent and these are what truly matter. We spend way too much time fixated on what the scale says. In reality, it has little importance. The scale can fluctuate daily, and this is demoralizing. Know that the scale may not reflect your success as accurately as assessing your body composition. Let go of your need to weigh or compare yourself based on what the scale reads. Look forward to changing your figure and not dealing with all the negative experiences that come from

BodyJoy Tip

Your weight on the scale can fluctuate on a daily basis. Water retention, time of day, elimination and other factors contribute to inconsistencies. When you starve yourself even one or two days you can lose 3-8 pounds, but your fat percent typically increases. The weight loss indicates a loss in muscle mass and water—NOT FAT. As soon as you eat or even take a drink, that scale can read a different number. Keep in mind the faster you lose weight, the faster you will put it back on! Concentrate on losing inches and body fat percent. Slow and steady is the way to go!

weighing. In fact, throw your scale away! Go ahead; I'll wait here for you.

Changing your body composition will bring you long-term results, not just in lost weight. Granted, your weight typically goes down when you lose fat and inches, but the extent of weight loss is different for everyone based on how much muscle you either maintain or gain. Did you know that muscle weighs more than fat, but it only takes up about one third the space?

I train a woman who recently retired. She began getting in more strength training, her sleep improved and her stress level decreased. After getting back into her smallest size clothing, she realized her weight was more than it was the previous time she wore the same clothing. Her body was getting smaller in terms of her inches, yet due to the fact she was increasing her muscle mass, the scale didn't go down as much as she was used to seeing. She was toning up and losing fat.

In the past when she lost weight, she starved herself and lost muscle mass so she weighed less. As a result, she could never keep the weight off. This time she weighed more, but lost several inches overall, was stronger, better toned and had great energy. The scale did not reflect her inch and body fat loss. She looked better than I had seen her (in over six years of training), her doctor said she was healthier and lowered several of her medicines, but she was not at her lowest weight.

For a while, this weight thing was frustrating to her. The scale was her main focus rather than the fact that she looked and felt her best. It was a long time between seeing her inches and fat decrease before her weight began to decrease. And once it began moving, the change was not as dramatic as her decrease in inches, body fat, and clothing sizes.

After getting accustomed to assessing her body fat and inches, my client began to feel excited about her improvements and hard work. In fact, she finally decided it doesn't matter what she weighs, as long as she continues changing her figure. It can be difficult to adjust to a new way of assessing your physical improvements but I know you can find pleasure and success at fitting into a smaller-size pant or having to go buy a smaller belt regardless of what the scale says!

In case you're interested here are some of her statistical measurements. The latest six-week Fitness Challenge this client participated in she lost eleven pounds (almost two pounds per week), which is a safe rate for weight loss. More impressively, she lost eighteen and a half inches overall and three percent body fat. Over the past six years, she has lost seventeen percent body fat, which has helped her finally fit into "regular" clothing sizes, no longer needing to shop in the "women's" section. She now bases her improvements on how her clothes fit, not her weight. You can tell in your pants and even the sleeves of your shirts if clothing is getting a little tighter than normal or if they are feeling roomier.

Begin to make assessments based on your clothing, even though weighing yourself is what you are accustomed to doing. Free yourself from the number fixation. What difference does it really make what you weigh if you look and feel better? Your weight may not correlate to dropping inches and clothing sizes the way you thought it should and that's okay. You can be your most fit and look your best regardless of what the scale says. It's time to pay attention to your body composition and forget about that number on the scale. If you didn't feel like you could do it the first time, here's your second chance . . . throw that scale away!

Commitment

Your success is related to your level of commitment. The biggest difference between my clients who achieve their goals versus those who don't is their level of commitment. It's not their schedule, financial situation, job, or family situation. These are all excuses.

Commitment is taking responsibility for your results. Commit to succeed. Decide you will make the time, be consistent, and remain focused towards achieving your goals. This time will be different because you will be committed.

The fact is *everyone* is *always* having to make an effort in terms of their fitness. It doesn't happen magically for people, it takes work and it isn't easy. It is attainable if you are willing to ACT on the things you learn and know. The concepts are basic, so you are going to figure out how to implement them and make them work for you in your body and life.

I heard someone once say that health and wellness is one of the best investments you can make. If you commit the time, effort and money now, your return will be ten-fold. It's one of the surest investments you'll ever find!

I am your personal trainer and life coach and these are the strategies you need to create the body and life you want. As your coach though, I turn the responsibility over to you. *You* are the expert in your life. Within you are all the answers you need to see results. With my guidance, YOU will create the results you desire. Your first assignment: Commit to not weighing yourself!

Strategy 2

Consistency

I have a client who used to restrict her calories to 800 per day for months at a time. She would go maybe three or four months and lose an average of 30 pounds (but her body fat would go up because she was losing muscle). Following the restrictive dieting months, she would find herself bingeing in a need to satisfy her cravings for the things she deprived herself of for so long. This client would train with me three months out of every year. Each year she would come back to me approximately 10 pounds heavier than from where she started the year before (prior to her severe calorie restricting phase). Over a four-year period she lost over 80 pounds, but ended up 20 pounds heavier than from where she originally started. She was the typical yo-yo dieter and emotional eater.

A few years ago she made a goal to end her over 40-year dieting cycle. She reframed her eating habits from emotional eating to eating for health and energy. She transitioned from rarely exercising to exercising on a daily basis. She began eating an appropriate amount of calories per day, having a variety of foods, eating whole foods more and less processed food choices (but not giving them up), and she consistently lost between 1-2 pounds a week for close to a year.

This time her fat percent continually decreased as well. She knew that if she remained consistent in her activity and maintained her calories at a level where she wasn't hungry and had energy, she'd continue to change her body and be able to maintain these changes once she achieved her final goal. She stopped dieting and she was losing weight, inches and body fat. This was the first time in her life she had felt full, had energy and understood her relationship with food.

It's been nearly two years since she began seeing results and she's continually striving towards her overall goal. She has dropped five clothing sizes so far. She continues to have more energy than before and receives compliments of how great she looks on a regular basis. Her inches and body fat percent are still decreasing each time we measure and she is much happier than I've ever seen her. Each month when we assess her progress, she has a great new story about how wonderful it felt to go have her clothes altered several inches or how glad she was to give away her biggest sized clothing. This client is in her mid 60s and she is living proof that you can make changes to your body at any stage of your life *if you are committed and consistent.*

Restrictions or quick fixes don't last. Rather than making drastic, unrealistic, dietary changes, make small improvements in your mindset, nutrition, and movement that will allow you to achieve long-term results. These are things you will incorporate into each day. Granted, achieving your goals the correct way takes longer than you may like, but it will create a new lifestyle that will provide consistency so you never have to fight the dieting battle again.

The way you change your body needs to mimic the way you maintain it—by consistency. If you will work on achieving your goals each and every day you'll find success. This isn't something you can work on for a month or six weeks then totally ignore. Make these efforts part of your life. Incorporate your goals into your lifestyle.

If you have a "bad eating day" forget about it the next day and begin to focus on your goal again. You won't make or break your success in one meal or one day of "bad eating". Learn why you made the decisions you did and take action to improve those actions the very next day.

Strategy 3

Environmental Factors

Willpower alone cannot compete with our "survival mode" wiring. And since we can't change our biology, we need to focus on an area where we do have control—our environment. Your environment can either make or break your success. To "make" your success, your environment must support what you are trying to achieve. If you are attempting to build new habits, be sure your environment doesn't resemble your old habits. Set yourself up for success.

For example, fill your kitchen or working environment with fruits, vegetables and whole grains. Avoid high-calorie, unhealthy processed foods when possible. Keep tempting processed treats out of sight or in a place you rarely look—not in your pantry or on your desk. Spend time with friends or family members who are active and who support you in your goals. Plan your day around finding ways to move so you burn calories even before or after your workout time. Keep in mind the other 23 hours of the day are just as important as that one hour you may spend exercising. Move as much as you can whenever you can.

Your environment was key to getting you where you are now, so in order to achieve the change you want, you must change your environment in a way that will support creating the new body you desire. Analyze your current environment. Is it consistent with what you are trying to achieve? Is it conducive for you to lose body fat, inches and reach your goals?

Does it support your efforts, or will it provide obstacles or roadblocks to your success? By changing your environment, you will create a path of less resistance and more fully ensure your success. Set yourself up to succeed!

It's right to make your environment personally comfortable, as well as conducive to success. If you still need a "treat" in the house, keep it—but move it out of sight. Surround yourself with whatever it is you need to succeed. This will be different for everyone, because we're all fueled by different stimuli.

Do what works for you and ignore the rest. If something hinders your success, change it! Keep improving your environment and you will keep improving yourself. Realistic, long-term results don't come by drastic changes, but by small improvements along the way. These changes replace old habits, and, soon become automatic. You truly are a product of your environment. Create an environment that will allow you to create your best self and experience body joy.

BodyJoy Tip

If you keep doing what you've always done, you'll keep getting what you've always got.

-    Peter Francisco

Our cultural environment is just as important as our home environment. We live in an age of unlimited technology (or so it seems). But, even though many things have made life more convenient, physically and emotionally, as a society we're heavier, unhappier and less fulfilled than ever before in history. Becoming healthier may mean taking a step back from some of the technology and modern convenience that's contributing to our inconvenient fat and excess inches.

Assess where technology may be hindering your goals. We rarely need to get up and move these days. If the TV remote is something you love, then find a different convenience to by-pass. I can live without having my car doors automatically open and shut. This makes me get up and move, especially on days I car pool. My driveway is relatively flat, so rather than snow blowing, I shovel our walks. I also prepare more meals using our dishes rather than using paper plates every night. I find I spend less time sitting on the couch and more time on my feet moving around before I sit. Small adjustments make a big difference in your figure.

There are a number of ways to make movement a larger part of our everyday routine if we don't allow modern conveniences to play a part in *everything* we do. I'm not saying shun it completely, just be conscious of the trade off. Just because technology has given you the opportunity to be motionless, doesn't mean you should.

I live just outside Salt Lake City. I use my car for transportation ninety percent of the time. When I travel to New York or other big cities, I walk for transportation and ninety percent of the time I come home with a lower body fat percentage and my clothes fitting looser. (Regardless of my New York dining experiences and less time spent in a gym.) I know that incorporating more walking into my day or moving more throughout my day helps improve my body. Although it's unreasonable to walk everywhere in my city, I have experimented with how to get a little more in where I can.

I walk next door to talk to my neighbors when possible. I take my dog out even for a few minutes if that is all the time I have. I play hide and seek, hiding on different levels of the house with my girls. I make several trips to the laundry room rather than piling up my baskets and going in one trip. I walk a few miles to take my girls to the park rather than going to the park on my street. I only bring in one bag of groceries from the car at a time when time permits. If time never permits for any of these small items, I reassess what I am doing and make time for at least some of them.

Pay attention to what helps you when you see any type of physical result. What small things have you noticed that work for you when you start to see an improvement? What additional trade offs could you incorporate on a regular basis that will work for you and your goals?

My mom is Canadian so growing up I spent countless summers in Magrath, Alberta, which is a tiny, simple, farm town. Although I am a city-girl, I loved how active and adventurous my days were on the Cook's farm. I would play to exhaustion; climbing trees, chasing around the animals, playing softball, swimming in the pond, fishing, taking the dogs out to be trained, feeding the animals, and hiking around the spill gates.

My Unc (who we stayed with) didn't stock a ton of treats in his house, so everyday my brothers and I walked three blocks to the candy store to buy something fun. (My favorite Canadian indulgence is the chocolate Nestle Smarties that you don't find in the US.) Even as a child, I could sense less stress in Magrath compared to Salt Lake and I enjoyed having that time to relax, play and recharge. We would go on daily walks to visit family friends. None of those things ever felt like exercise. They were just activities that were part of each day during our visit in Canada.

I also noticed a wonderful difference between the tastes of fresh, farm-grown food, versus the processed counter parts I typically ate. I spent most of my vacations picking and eating all the sugar snap peas in my great-uncle's garden. I filled up on fresh carrots, peas and tomatoes, consuming more vegetable than I typically ate at home.

All produce does not taste the same! There is something more rich, flavorful and enjoyable about fresh whole foods. I was just recently reminded of it again last summer as I had the opportunity to visit the Cook's farm and take my husband and girls. I was reminded that lunchtime was always the largest meal on the farm.

Most American's have dinner as their largest meal. I've tried to do a better job incorporating a large lunch into my days so I have more energy to help me with my activities and less calories to burn off in the evening time. This also helps me avoid binging after work or in the evenings.

Another observation I made was how fit and lean the farmers still are. They were always trim and fit when I was a little girl and 30 years later they continue to be healthy, lean and strong. A farm way of life is unrealistic for me and maybe for you, but incorporating some of these farm habits can help create a stronger, leaner body.

Eat larger portions earlier in the day when your demand for energy is high. Plant a garden or shop the farmer's markets so you can experience the pleasure of fresh vegetables. I love shopping the farmer's markets in the fall and try to buy as fresh of food as possible. In the winter, my farmer's market sells fresh apple juice and preserves. It may mean more frequent trips to the grocery store or an extra trip to the farmer's market, but they are well worth it!

I have a girlfriend who is from Italy named Gaia. She moved to the United States a few years ago and I have learned so many healthy concepts from her European habits and lifestyle. She eats mostly whole foods and very little processed foods. This is just the way she was raised. She was even making her own pasta for a while.

As an American, with very different lifestyle habits (who had never experienced fresh pasta) I questioned her sanity. Gaia has an amazing appetite and an even more amazing figure, so I've paid attention to what she does in terms of cooking and eating. Gaia's food is unlike any food I've ever tasted. (My parents are both excellent cooks by the way!) Gaia introduced me to the difference in flavor using fresh herbs versus dried.

I have also gained a greater appreciation for eating more variety of fresh vegetables compared to my usual routine. She adds fresh vegetables into so many dishes. She's proof that eating mainly whole foods that taste amazing and only processed foods on occasion produce quite different results in terms of weight and inches.

Gaia recently returned from visiting her mom in Rome. She commented on how few buildings in Italy actually have elevators or escalators. She forgot how much walking and climbing stairs she did back home. Since most American's live in much younger cities and with ADA building code regulations, nearly every building higher than one story has an elevator or escalator. How often do you take the stairs? This is one of the conveniences that I try and bypass when I can. No matter how fit you are, there is nothing like a staircase workout, even if you're just walking up them. What a wonderfully effective, no-hassle way to incorporate more movement into your day.

I have a client named Vicki who grew up on a farm and is a talented gardener. She has brought me fresh produce from her garden and has helped me realize the pleasure in eating seasonally. She is my consultant on which time of year to try different vegetables and fruits. Even though most everything is available to us year round in our grocery stores, an apple in February just doesn't taste the same as it does in high season. Different times of year can produce different varieties of foods to enjoy. The variety keeps us from getting board with the same old foods, making us healthier and more satisfied.

I've also discovered I need to enjoy seasonal processed treats "seasonally" as well. For Christmas, my friend John makes English toffee I anticipate the entire year. I savor each piece knowing it will be 11 more months until I enjoy it again. (It's a good thing I don't have it available year-round.) I get so excited around Easter time when the grocery stores stock Cadbury Mini-Eggs. These were once my downfall, buying bags galore during the season and trying to stretch them out year round.

Only, that plan backfired as I devoured all the bags within the month of April. Now I eat seasonal processed foods more sensibly. I only buy one bag a year of the Cadbury Mini-Eggs and know when they're gone, that's it for the season. I enjoy and savor them more than I did eating unlimited amounts and I find that my bathing suits still fit in time for summer this way.

The anticipation can be part of the experience of enjoying the treat. I reserve fondue for only two special occasions each year. I only bring home donuts on Halloween. (Yes, that means once a year!) I buy Halloween candy the day before trick-or-treating so I don't eat an entire bag on my own. My girls are permitted to eat two pieces of candy a day until their Halloween or Valentine's candy is gone and we keep it up in our Tupperware cabinet, not the pantry where we see it often.

As you read through this book, take inventory on which concepts or ideas may be a natural fit for you. Nothing needs to be extreme or overly restrictive. If something feels too tough, adapt it to what seems manageable or doable. Don't be afraid to try new ideas. Evaluate others around you who seem to be fit and healthy. Pay attention to their lifestyle habits or their rituals. Dave, the swim director at my gym has an amazing physique.

Gym members constantly ask me how he eats and what he does in the weight room to look as fit as he does. Dave is over 50 and has the chiseled, lean body most 30 year olds never achieve. What they forget is his healthy nutrition and weight room activity are just two aspects contributing to his figure. In addition to his whole foods nutrition and weights, Dave swims miles on a daily basis, bikes to and from work, hikes regularly, and is extremely active throughout his day, not just the hour he spends in the weight room.

In addition to those around you, observe other cultures that seem to have wellness and health just happen as a result of their daily habits. Meditation, less processed foods and regular movement has created healthy societies. Get inspiration from wherever it presents itself. Anything to contribute to a healthier environment, both culturally and at home will help you reach your goals.

BodyJoy Tip

Eat your favorite and seasonal treats, but find a healthier fashion in how you enjoy them and know there will be more to enjoy for seasons to come.

What are some steps you can take to create a supportive environment?

_____

_____

_____

_____

_____

_____

_____

_____

_____

_____

_____

_____

_____

_____

_____

_____

_____

_____

_____

_____

You can refer to my Healthy Tips section for additional ideas and add to this as you progress through the book. We've only scratched the surface!

Strategy 4

Overcoming "Bad Body Days" by
Discovering Your Body Type

"What a disgrace for a man to grow old without ever seeing the beauty and grace of which his body is capable."

—Socrates

Often when setting goals for changing our bodies, we compare ourselves to the supermodels on TV, or perhaps our friend with the "perfect" body. Countless times, I have had new training clients come into their first session asking to look like the person in a magazine picture. Some people have requested my services because I train their friend or someone else they know and they want to look just the way that person does. I have women regularly asking me how to get legs like the Victoria Secret models and men inquiring how to develop abs like the bodybuilders or some other person's body that they admire.

Did you know that most of the models don't even look the way they do in ads? The beautiful actress Kate Winslet demonstrated this by revealing in an interview that her cover shot for *GQ Magazine* was extensively, digitally enhanced to where her legs ended up looking only half the size they truly are.

The cultural pressure to look a certain way is overwhelming. Attractiveness is defined by narrow, unattainable stereotypes. The reality of it is that most of us could never achieve the expectations we set on our body simply because we're not built that way. It's unrealistic for you to compare your individual shape to those of another category, but I bet you do it sometimes!

I spent all of my teenage years and the first part of my twenties wanting to look like my beautiful friends who were all at least 5'8" tall with long limbs and flat stomachs. It took me thousands of dollars spent with my personal trainer and many frustrating hours for him to convince me I could be just as beautiful and fit at 5'4", but I could not and never would look like my girlfriends because I had a different body type.

Unfortunately, most of us don't have the genetic build to be supermodels or look like bodybuilders. However, all body types do have the potential to be healthy, fit and attractive. An important fact to keep in mind is that losing inches and body fat will not change your genetic build or body type. Regardless of what shape you are, you do have the ability to improve your figure to its fullest potential. Stop comparing yourself to others and work on being the best *you* can become.

There are three specific body types and variations within each specific type. Recognize which category you fall into and know that whichever shape you have, you can make physical improvements. The three distinct body types are ectomorph, mesomorph and endomorph.

Mesomorphs are muscular, broad shouldered, and thick-chested. Individuals with this body type tend to store excess fat in their stomach region, increasing their risks of heart disease, cancers and type II diabetes. This is the body type that notably is associated with the "beer" belly—even if they aren't drinkers. The abdominal region is where these people typically gain body fat before it is noticeable in other locations.

Endomorphs are rounder overall and more pear shaped. These individuals tend to store fat around the hips, butt and thighs, increasing their risk of obesity and joint issues. This is where I fit in! The first place I start to see an increase when I gain body fat is in my thighs and rear. It's also the last place I experience improvements when I am working on my goals.

Ectomorphs are typically tall and slender. These body types are the people you hear complaining about how hard it is to gain muscle and increase size. My girlfriends fall into this category and so does my husband. My husband has spent his entire life trying to increase his size. It took him the first nine years of our marriage to put on 12 pounds of muscle and maintain it. (My body type can gain 10 pounds in two weeks! The only thing is that it wouldn't be muscle!) When we vacation for a few days or if he isn't lifting weights regularly, he ends up losing weight without even trying.

This is the body type most of us compare ourselves to. I can't imagine losing mass on vacation. If I'm not conscious of my activity and eating, I tend to gain it! It's just as hard for ectomorphs to gain muscle or lean mass as it is for mesomorphs and endomorphs to lose body fat.

Each specific body type has its challenges and unique ability to look appealing.

Which body type do you fit into? _____

BodyJoy Tip

Obesity is now the second highest killer of Americans, according to Center for Disease Control statistics. A loss of only 19% of your body weight is enough to decrease high blood pressure, lower cholesterol and triglycerides, and improve your overall medical health.

Regardless of your body type, appreciate the body you've been given[1]:

- Celebrate yourself! You are unique.
- Identify your positive features and appreciate them.
- Enjoy living actively.
- Try a new physical activity. Move each day just because it feels good.
- Realize that fitness and nutrition (not your weight) are the keys to adding healthy years to your life.
- Get your family and friends involved in being active. Doing something together is always more fun!
- Accept, respect and celebrate people of different sizes, shapes, ethnic backgrounds, abilities and talents.

---

[1] *Adapted from HealthyHabits.com*

- Think critically when looking at media images and messages. Are they realistic and supportive of a healthy lifestyle?
- Take time every day to nurture yourself in some way.
- Stay in tune with your body.
- Help others feel good about themselves and who they are.
- Take what works for you and throw out the rest!
- Trust your ability to make choices to better your health.
- Wear clothes that are comfortable and that make you feel good. Work with your body, not against it.
- Do something for your body to let it know you appreciate it—take a bath, nap or find some time to relax outdoors.
- Your goals should include becoming the best *you* that you can be.

List five things you like about yourself that do not relate to your weight or what you look like:

1. _____

2. _____

3. _____

4. _____

5. _____

BodyJoy Tip

Treat yourself with respect. Like what you see in the mirror everyday and focus on living well, not just looking good.

Strategy 5

The BodyJoy Body Image: Self-Respect

The sixties introduced super-thin twiggy models, fad diets and weight-loss centers. Today, underweight models are considered beautiful and there are more fad diets and weight-loss centers than ever before. Society seems to have accepted a very narrow definition of beauty, which has resulted in more eating disorders, higher levels of depression and lowered self-respect. Obesity and eating disorders have reached epidemic levels. It's hard not to get sucked in. We have all had bad body days!

Since body image and happiness are directly related, it's essential for you to find body confidence and self-acceptance no matter what size you are. You can have a good body image and be happy now even though you are trying to improve your figure, health and fitness. Honest appreciation of your body with all its strengths and weaknesses is essential. How do you do that? By being at peace with your life, either accepting it or changing it to where you would like it to be. This is an important element for experiencing BodyJoy.

Body image is about how satisfied you are with your life—feelings about yourself, relationships, and your situation. Your body image reflects and affects your self-respect and feelings of self-worth. Self-respect begins internally. It's a higher feeling of esteem that you hold for yourself. It's displayed in thoughts and actions. Insist on treating yourself with positive thoughts, language, actions and feelings, and insist that others respond to you in the same fashion. In turn, treat others this way. It's a golden rule of life—treat others as you would have them treat you.

How you feel about yourself has much more of an impact than how others view you. You will struggle with BodyJoy if you let your self-respect be governed by others' opinions or if you are fixated on the numbers that show on your scale. Having solid self-respect allows all aspects of your life to fall into place and makes setbacks seem less overwhelming. Strong self-respect begins with working on your mind and your body.

How do you view your body?
Describe your body.

_____
_____
_____
_____
_____
_____
_____

Which adjectives did you use? Did you scrutinize specific areas or did you describe what your body is capable of doing? Do you see it as a passive object or do you view your body as having a purpose and see it as something active?

Your body is an amazing gift to be used in a number of ways. When you are using your body for a purpose, weight loss and a flat stomach tend to take care of themselves. When you are moving and using your body to accomplish goals and tasks, you can improve your health, figure and weight. Your focus can be on your accomplishments, not just on your shape.

When you view your body as something active it's easier to concentrate on your health and how you feel. Do you focus on your health and how you feel or are you sacrificing feeling good about yourself by obsessing over your weight? Are you starving, bingeing, feeling tired, short-tempered, sad or bored? Self-respect is an experience. It's a particular way of experiencing yourself. It's more than a mere feeling. It involves emotional, evaluative, and cognitive components. It also entails certain action dispositions: to move toward life rather than away from it, to treat facts about your body and life with respect rather than denial, and to function responsibly.

If you lack self-respect, it will be difficult to find happiness, peace, and BodyJoy, even in your "ideal" body. I trained one particular client that appeared to have it all. This woman was beautiful, thin, and toned. She was the person everyone in the gym wanted to look like. Unfortunately her interior didn't reflect her exterior.

She was essentially unhappy, unsure, and insecure. She compared herself to everyone around her, being compulsive about her weight and extremely obsessive about each little section of her body. She fought depression and dealt with these issues by abusing both prescription and illegal drugs. From the outside she looked perfect and appeared basically happy, but inside she didn't feel anything like she looked.

As her trainer, my goal for her was to find some peace of mind and self-respect, alongside of her physical goals. After she figured out her way of "existing" was not a fulfilling way to live, I recommended she seek out help from a professional therapist. She tried a few different people and began seeing a holistic therapist. She "cleared" some of her internal issues so she could be a solid person internally as well as what her body projected.

There are various types of therapy that can effectively help resolve issues related to poor self-respect. Different methods work for different people. If necessary, seek out these avenues to help you reach your health and fitness goals. You don't have to conquer them by yourself. With my client, there was a noticeable difference in her attitude, self-respect and behavior while she was going through her sessions. I witnessed her transform into a happier, self-confident, in-control person.

She treats herself better and expects that same level of respect from those around her. She can now appreciate her body and she honors its limitations, rather than searching for happiness based on how defined her abs were or how thin she could become. Transforming your level of self-respect is important for you to experience before you're able to transform your body.

Self-respect is the disposition to experience yourself as being competent to cope with the basic challenges of life and of being worthy of happiness. Self-respect means having unconditional self-acceptance regardless of what you do or don't do. It means having confidence in your decisions and in your ability to think.

It is confidence in your ability to learn, to make appropriate choices and decisions, and to respond effectively to change. It is also the experience that you are entitled to success, achievement, fulfillment, and happiness.[2] Self-respect can help you take control of your body. It can allow you to be responsible and accountable for your experiences and your results.

Lack of self-respect, dieting and obsessing about the scale, tends to bring on a number of negative thoughts and feelings. Do you know you have wonderful qualities because you are you—not because of your shape or your size?

Describe your life. What is it like? How does it make you feel?

_____
_____
_____
_____
_____
_____

BodyJoy Tip

Looking good and having a positive body image is not vanity; it is your road to a long, healthy, and happy life.

- Dr. Nicolas Perricone, *The Perricone Promise*

If you are like most typical Americans, you probably described your life as stressed, tiring, lacking time, crazy, busy, and on-the-go. I would love for you to be able to list fulfilling, happy and satisfied, at peace, energetic, eventful, challenging, rewarding and blessed.

Until you are at peace with your inner self you won't find success with your outer self. Happiness doesn't come once the scale reads a certain number. I have countless clients who can attest to this! I've seen people reach their physical goals and still be unhappy and I have witnessed people become happy and fulfilled regardless of their size. Are you secure with your life and your situation? Happiness can come from taking care of you, being less critical, and avoiding competition or comparisons. These only worsen insecurities.

---

[2] *Association for Self-Esteem website, www.self-esteem-nase.org*

Sometimes you may feel like you don't have time or can't afford to focus on yourself since there are so many others you need to concentrate on (family members, friends, co-workers, etc.). Focusing on being your best you is not a selfish thing. When you are at your best, you are better able to take care of others and help them achieve their wants and needs.

You can be a better support and greater example when you emulate happiness, peace and health. You are less of a burden to those you care about when you are healthy and active. You can achieve this at any age.

Your self-respect affects the way you think and feel about yourself. Do you know the body will obey the mind? You have the power to change your perceptions, your body, your ability to be happy, full of joy and at peace. The body is designed to be healthy and fit. By taking responsibility for

BodyJoy Tip

The precondition for happiness with others is a good relationship with yourself. This means respecting yourself, being an adult and meeting your own needs, finding love with yourself first; then family, friends, co-workers, acquaintances and the world.

how you feel and think, you can determine your success. Balance taking care of your mental and physical needs and wants to help find peace with yourself, your body, and your life.

Ways to Improve your Body Image, Happiness and Self-Respect

- Try new activities.
- Play.
- Use your body for accomplishing something rather than as something to be looked at. Do a walk for charity, climb a mountain or go on a hike, enter a 5-k, 10-k, or marathon, a triathlon, or any other event.
- Meditate, do yoga, and stretch.
- Don't allow others or yourself to negatively label you.
- Get involved in a cause or serve others to put things into perspective.

- Practice good posture.
- Care more about how you feel rather than what others may be thinking of how you look.
- Don't compare yourself to anyone except yourself.
- Don't allow others to suck you into their negative attitudes.
- Examine your attitudes, beliefs, prejudices and behaviors about food, weight, body image, physical appearance, health and exercise.
- Despite media and social pressure, know that weight and appearance are not the most important indicators of your identity and self-worth.
- Decide which internal values are important to you and focus on them, such as compassion, sympathy, wisdom, loyalty, fairness, self-respect, self-worth, confidence, individuality, ambition, motivation, sense of humor, and respect.
- Respect and accept others for who they are.
- Love and respect yourself, your body and your achievements.
- Nurture yourself first, so you can give to others without depleting your energy.
- Find ways to be happy.
- Focus on the positive.
- Love who you are.

Your sense of competence and self-respect can be strengthened through realistic and accurate self-appraisal, meaningful accomplishments, overcoming adversities, bouncing back from failures, and assuming responsibility and maintaining integrity.[3] Don't waste another moment being critical of yourself. Focus on your qualities and gifts and watch how much easier it is for you to achieve your goals. Play off your strengths. Go back and read or add to the list of things you like about yourself.

---

[3]   *Adapted from Association for Self-Esteem website, www.self-esteem-nase.org, THE TRUE MEANING OF SELF-ESTEEM by Robert Reasoner*

Strategy 6

The BodyJoy Approach: Positive Thinking,

Positive Language, Positive Perception

A simple shift in thinking is what you need to go from an unhealthy or unfit body to your goal body. Approach this new plan with a positive attitude. You will not be asked to completely stop eating anything you love or to exercise to exhaustion. You will only being asked to change or modify the way you're doing some things now.

After all, a large portion of this plan is having you experience joy! Change will be easier if you replace an old habit with a new one that you enjoy and that you know will make you feel better about yourself. This is not about all or nothing! You won't miss cutting back on certain foods because you'll have alternative foods to fill their place. **Adapting your focus from what you can't have all the time to what you are entitled to will make a drastic difference in your level of success.** Think entitlement! You are entitled to live your best life in your best body.

BodyJoy Tip

If you believe you can, you can. If you believe you can't, you're probably right.

—Anonymous

One of my favorite "pearls of wisdom" is that we should treat others according to their potential, not according to how they are. Apply this to yourself. Treat yourself as if you're at your ideal body size. Treat yourself as a fit, healthy, and active person. Feel the happiness, peace and health you will enjoy in your goal body. Get into the positive mindset of success.

Have you ever heard of the Law of Attraction? Simply put, the Law of Attraction is that whatever you put your attention on, in belief, thought and feeling, it will come into your life. This Law works similarly to how a magnet works. When a metal object is near a magnet, it's naturally drawn to it. The object has no choice but to be pulled toward the magnet.

Whatever we are focused on or whatever occupies our thoughts is what we attract or create. There is no exclusion in the Law of Attraction, so if you're constantly thinking about what you don't want, then that's what you'll end up getting.

Those of us who have dieted have experienced the Law of Attraction—even though we may not have recognized it. We obsess about what the scale says and what we cannot have. We deprive ourselves of food—yet what we are not supposed to be eating is all we think about. We are obsessed with not gaining weight and we worry whether or not we're losing any pounds. We end up focusing so much on what we cannot or should not have and do, that we end up bingeing and sabotaging our own efforts.

Look at how successful you have been at attracting what you don't want. Imagine how successful you could be at attracting what you really want if your focus were in the right direction. Your beliefs or perceptions create your experience. Changing your perception from deprivation to entitlement can free you from being stuck with what you don't want. One of the greatest powers we have is the ability to change our perception—to take something that's overwhelming and make it manageable or less of an obstacle, such as food. Your mind responds the same whether it's actual or merely a perception.

BodyJoy Tip

"O" Magazine's January 2005 issue had this wonderful quote on its monthly calendar. "Make 'I can' an integral part of your vocabulary. Whenever you're tempted to say 'I can't', stop, take a deep breath, and imagine what would happen if you gave it your all."

I have a neighbor who's a psychologist. He taught me that psychologists use the *ABC Model* to illustrate how influential your perception is as well. Say you have an *Arbitrary Event* or situation such as being overweight or needing to lose "x" amount of inches. Your *Beliefs (perceptions and thoughts)* lead to your *Consequences* or outcomes and results. So if you're overweight and you believe you will always be heavy, or that you will never be able to lose excess body fat, then these are the consequences you're likely to receive.

Not only your beliefs, but your language, self-talk, thoughts and perceptions affect your feelings and the behaviors that result as consequences. For example, you might feel as if you're not worth it, you may not like yourself, you may be depressed, you may think others don't like you and you may be unhappy with yourself and those around you. You may eat to console yourself or out of hopelessness that you will ever be able to change.

If you can change your beliefs or perception from hopelessness or feeling that you'll never be able to change to feeling that you *can* change, you will begin to see different consequences or results. When you shift your beliefs from what you *can't* do to what you *can* do or what you *want* to have happen, you unleash the potential to generate positive feelings and behaviors that can in turn create or attract the results you desire. You can take your body from survival mode to thriving.

I was skeptical when I first read that positive thoughts can lead to success. Then I met a woman who attributed her 20-pound weight loss to standing in front of the mirror and repeating positive affirmations. This was the only conscious change she made to her lifestyle—it didn't directly deal with eating or exercising. As a personal trainer I knew changing a person's body had to do with burning calories and eating less, not standing in front of the mirror, but the more I learned how powerful positive perceptions are, the more I recognized they can be an essential key in changing bodies and minds.

In fact, this was the missing element for me as I was struggling to find my best body. During my journey to finding body joy I was exercising. I was watching my nutrition. I was trying to lose body fat and inches, but was focusing on how I looked and my "problem areas," not on how I wanted to look or what I could achieve.

It wasn't until I refocused my attention on what I wanted (not where I was), that my efforts started to produce results. My perception was keeping me stuck in many negative habits. When you improve your state of mind, you can improve your habits, which can lead to changing and improving your body. Positive language and thoughts can fuel your efforts and help you reach your goals.

Decide now. What *do* you want? You are literally creating your own world around you with your thoughts, beliefs, language and perceptions. You can have or create whatever you want. Just like the woman I met, you too can lose 20 pounds or achieve whatever your goal is with the help of a positive perception. Her positive perception allowed other elements to fall into place so she could take the measures necessary to reach her goal. If you don't like what you're experiencing, change your thoughts now! Choose to *act* rather than *react* to your situation.

Your future will be determined by whatever thoughts and beliefs you are currently having and what you continue to believe. If you think and worry about what you don't want, believing it's a way to protect or safeguard yourself, you are fooling yourself. Look at the success you've had up until now! The best way to give yourself what you do want is to imagine it, get excited about it, allow it to happen, and then express gratitude when it does come.

BodyJoy Tip

The present is the future you envisioned for yourself long ago. Let the choices you make today be choices you want to live with tomorrow.

"I am" are two of the most powerful words in our vocabulary. When you say, "I am," you are creating your present reality. By saying "I am," in reference to things you don't want in your life such as "I am fat, I am ugly, I am sick and tired, I am unhappy, I am worthless," you put more attention on the negative and create more of what you don't want.[4]

Start right now imagining your life and body exactly how you want it to be. How big can you dream? How much joy can you hold? Your intention to feel good and be healthy and fit will be honored and your body can start

---

4   *Tuttle, Carol, Remembering Wholeness, Elton-Wolf Publishing, Seattle, WA, 2003,* *www.caroltuttle.com*

to change. Reprogram your language and self-talk from negative thoughts into positive ones. Refer to the following list for ideas.

Positive Thoughts

- I am healthy.
- I am thin.
- I am fit.
- I am losing inches.
- I look good.
- I feel good.
- I am creating a better body.
- I am grateful for my healthy body.
- I am experiencing more energy and vitality.
- I am successful.
- I am deserving.
- I am comfortable with my body.
- I am grateful to be alive.
- I am happy.
- I am free from food cravings.
- I am using food properly.
- I am enjoying exercise.
- I want others to feel good just being around me.
- I feel good when I move.
- I enjoy exercising regularly.
- I am beautiful.
- I am strong.
- I am worth it.
- I am achieving my goals.
- I look great.
- I am successful.
- I can do it.
- I am at peace with myself.
- I enjoy moving.
- I am experiencing BodyJoy.

How to Implement Positive Language, Thoughts and Perceptions

Copy some of these statements and hang them where you can read some or all of them every day. Repeat these thoughts to yourself on a regular basis. Think positive thoughts as often as you can. It will become your reality. When you catch yourself drifting into the negative, remember how powerful your positive thoughts can be. Change your "I can't" into "I can". Your thoughts are key to your future success.

Imagine how you would like to look and feel. Close your eyes and literally see yourself at your desired size, health, or fitness level as you go through the list of affirmations above. Create your own thoughts or statements in addition to those provided. Start with a few positive thoughts that work for you, and then incorporate more once you feel comfortable with them. These statements will become part of your life, helping you create a new and more enjoyable experience.

Start talking nice to yourself. Stop apologizing, justifying, defending, and explaining yourself. Know you are worthy of your own respect. Start esteeming yourself in your thoughts and actions. Be aware of things you do that weaken your self-respect and take action to change them. If you criticize, judge and condemn yourself, begin to let go of those mental habits. Incorporate new mental habits of positive language and unconditional self-acceptance.

Avoid putting other people down. Validate, validate, validate! This is the greatest way to build self-respect in others and yourself. Validate how much you love yourself and those around you, validate their feelings, validate the idea that there is nothing they have to do to be loved by you. Validate that you are worth the time and effort you are taking to improve your body and mind. It starts with one simple thought of encouragement!

Take baby steps to mentally engrain positive language and thoughts. Each week write down two positive statements, either ones you have thought of or statements from the list provided. Write them on a sticky note or note card and put it where you will regularly see it. Hang it on your bathroom mirror, on the dashboard in your car, on your computer monitor, or on the fridge. Make a point to read the statements or recite them to yourself often throughout the day. The following week, add two more statements to your list and begin repeating the new statements to yourself. Soon positive self-talk will be automatic and it will be easy for you to come up with new statements.

A common time for me to practice positive self-talk is whenever I start to get frustrated, especially when I am training for a marathon or when one of my workouts gets tough. When I'm on a long run and my body begins to feel tired or my muscles feel uncomfortable, I consciously change my focus. I begin focusing on how far I have come, how good I felt my first few miles, and how good it feels to finish a run.

I feel grateful for the ability I have to push my body, that it will take me where I need it to and that it allows me to experience what I feel when I accomplish a distance run or race. Believe me; the right perception can get you through almost anything. I know it can make a difference in your success!

Confront Your Fears

Fear is one of the many emotions we experience. It has its purpose just like all other emotions. Fear protects us from danger. However, most people are conditioned to fear situations that are not life threatening and, due to our habituated responses, we treat many everyday situations as such. In this case, fear is a distracting negative emotion.

BodyJoy Tip

"Our deepest fear is not that we are inadequate. Our deepest fear is that we are powerful beyond measure. It is our light, not our darkness, that most frightens us. We ask ourselves, Who am I to be brilliant, gorgeous, talented, fabulous? Actually, who are you not to be? You are a child of God. Your playing small doesn't serve the world. There's nothing enlightened about shrinking so that other people won't feel insecure around you. We were born to make manifest the glory of God that is within us. It's not just in some of us; it's in everyone. And as we let our own light shine, we unconsciously give other people permission to do the same. As we're liberated from our own fear, our presence automatically liberates others."

- *Marianne Williamson*

Many fears are inherent within us, while others are self-taught. It's an emotion that comes up for many people as they begin to think about changing their body or life. Perhaps it has been an obstacle in keeping you stuck with the results you have experienced in the past.

Today, create a fear list, journaling about all the things you are afraid of that relate to improving your body, health or fitness. Then decide whether they are worth the energy you devote to thinking about them. If not, decide instead to focus on things you love or things that will enhance a positive perception. Don't spend any more time being victim to negative thoughts and feelings. Change your perception so you can experience positive results.

Fear List

_____
_____
_____
_____
_____
_____
_____

I regularly try to replace fear with gratitude. It drastically alters my focus from the negative to thinking positive. I use the time I spend walking my dog or taking my girls in the baby jogger to think of all the things I have to be grateful for. I keep a notebook in our kitchen and when it's out on the table, my family thinks of things that we're grateful for and we add these things to our gratitude list. We play the "gratitude game" in the car when my girls get anxious or restless. We take turns saying what each of us is grateful for, seeing how long we can go before something is repeated.

Gratitude and love can be a stronger emotion than fear if you get into the habit of focusing positive. Believe it or not, all of these "mental" issues contribute to losing fat and inches. They create your state of mind and your ability to create a new, better experience. On the other hand, these issues have the power to keep you trapped in the same cycle you've experienced up until now.

BodyJoy Tip

"Put love first. Entertain thoughts that give life. And, when a thought of resentment, or hurt, or fear comes your way have another thought that is more powerful—a thought that is love."

- Mary Manin Morrissey

Whether it's improving your perception, language, and self-talk, or better understanding what gives you the initiative to eat better, move more and experience body joy; you need to take whatever steps are necessary for _you_ to achieve your goals. Don't wait until you've finished this book, but start today.

Strategy 7

Identify Your Eating Behavior

"Behavioral and environmental factors are large contributors to overweight and obesity and provide the greatest opportunity for actions and interventions designed for prevention and treatment."

—*Surgeon General's Call to Action on Obesity*

Finding your best body isn't about following a strictly written "diet" plan. Generally, you know which foods are the healthiest choices. Finding your best body is about recognizing your triggers and understanding *what* sends you to the fridge or pantry or *why* you're eating when you do. All the nutritional information in the world won't do a bit of good if you don't understand your eating type or *why* you eat. This is why despite the best intentions; many individuals trying to change their figures are not successful over the long-term. Unfortunately, most of them blame themselves and their lack of willpower rather than considering important lifestyle and behavioral factors.

These factors can include how you feel about your body, your goals, and your dieting history. Before you set your goals, it's important to consider *why* you eat. This will help you discover which factors are issues that may impact your success. After all, losing body fat and inches is not just about burning calories: it's about your relationship to food. It's important to have a peaceful relationship with food to successfully reach your goals.

Which type of eater do you think you are?[5]

Careful/"Good" Eater

To an outsider you appear to be very health conscious, disciplined and in control. Instead of enjoying food and the nourishment it gives your body, you may find yourself analyzing every mouthful for its effect on your body, its health benefits and the calories it represents. You tend to classify food as either "good" or "bad", "safe" or "unsafe". Does this sound like you?

Nighttime Eater

Many Americans (especially over-extended women) fit into this category. Diet-minded individuals are classic "nighttime eaters" as well. Do you think you are doing "so good" if you hardly eat any calories in the day? Do you start your day by skipping breakfast or with a cup of coffee or soda? Do you have a meal replacement bar for lunch (if you have time) and then find yourself starving by 4 p.m.? Do you munch on "treat foods" once you begin eating and really have no idea how much food you consume?

If so, you are probably a "nighttime eater". Without fuel throughout the day, your body cannot run as strongly or efficiently. By nighttime, you feel as if you "deserve" to eat what you want, or since you are uncontrollably hungry, you go for it. Not because you want to, but because you give in to cravings since you're depleted and starving. You tend to eat the majority of your calories when you're more sedentary and need less fuel. Does this sound like you?

"As Much as Possible before Monday Morning" Eater

This is the sign of a classic dieter! You eat as much as possible during the weekend, with the idea that Monday will be the start of a new diet (again). This usually backfires by Wednesday and the whole cycle continues over

---

[5]   *Adapted from Beth Wolfgram, CSCS, MS, RD, CD, www.bethwolfgram.com and Intuitive Eating by Evelyn Tribole and Elyse Resch, ISBN 0312321236.*

and over and over. You move to restrictive thinking. You say you'll never eat that way again and you blame yourself or think, "What's wrong with me since I can't keep on this diet?" Does this sound like you?

Emotional Eater

Who hasn't used food at some point to feel better? It is easy for most overweight people to relate to this category. If you find yourself continually using food when you are happy, angry, sad, frustrated, stressed or disappointed, then most likely you are an emotional eater. Emotional triggers often send you looking for food to help you cope with your emotions, pressures, stresses, and daily life. Does this sound like you?

On-the-Run Eater

Your life is overscheduled and you always feel crazed. You don't have time to cook or prepare meals, so you eat out frequently. You find yourself eating in your car, at your desk, or while waiting in line. You probably find your eating patterns to be haphazard and sporadic. Does this sound like you?

Intuitive Eater

Eating intuitively means you honor your hunger. You eat when you are hungry and stop when you are no longer hungry. You enjoy food for the taste and nourishment, without guilt or resentment. You eat to fuel your body or to have energy sufficient to accomplish activities at hand. Does this sound like you?

Which Type of Eater are you?

_____

You may have seen yourself in more than one of these categories—that's normal! If you found that the majority of your eating is done regardless of intuition, or honoring your hunger or satiety (feeling of being full), you need to refocus and remember one of the primary purposes you need food for is FUEL.

When you approach food as a form of fuel, rather than as a past-time or source of comfort, it is easier to break the bond that it may have on you. Food is an essential part of your survival. You need it to thrive. Food is your primary source of energy; it is neither good nor bad, it is food. Food is neutral. Habits pertaining to how and why you eat food may be considered "bad" habits or "poor" choices, but these habits can be changed and improved. In order for you to concentrate on food as a fuel source, abandon dieting and learn to listen to your body.

"Normal" eating occurs when you listen to the internal signals of hunger, satiety and appetite. You eat when you are hungry and stop when you are satisfied. (This is not completely full or stuffed!) Normal eating keeps your body from feeling starved or overly stuffed. It's a state of contentment. For most people, this means eating between four and eight times daily. When you don't listen to your body, you may overeat or under eat. This often leads to fasting, skipping meals, bingeing, dieting and eating for emotional reasons.

Being able to listen to your body is the key to finding optimal health and your ideal size. Many individuals eat for reasons other than hunger. By listening to your internal signals you can eat for health, gain energy and eat with pleasure and enjoyment. When you are in tune with your body's needs, food choices tend to be more varied and balanced. You can more successfully attend to other issues that may be calling for your attention when you are aware they may not be related to food hunger.

Strategy 8

Overcoming Behavioral Eating

As you've read, food is used for much more than as a source of nourishment. Behavioral eating can become a replacement for self-respect and is representative of losing control over the body. Some negative or what you may view as "bad" nutrition habits stem from a lack of unfulfilled needs or desires. Food is used to cope with these issues, but in actuality we need something other than food. Sometimes they are merely a reflection of unawareness or poor planning. Here are some suggestions to combat behavioral eating.

Careful/"Good" Eater

If healthy nutrition basics are followed, you do not need to worry about counting calories religiously or making sure you're getting all of the required nutrients. If you're trying to control your intake of a substance, even if that substance is food, you have to take your focus off it, or you'll only be fueling your obsession and sabotaging your efforts. Moderation can be practiced better when food is not obsessively organized. By changing the emphasis from what you cannot have and focusing on the foods that are healthy for you, you shouldn't need to stress about every single thing you eat. Food does not need to consume your every thought and action.

This was my eating type when I traveled as a marketing executive. When I went on a business trip, I took as much food with me as clothes. I was constantly thinking about when I needed to eat, what I was going to eat, and if the foods I enjoyed would be available at the different restaurants. Food occupied my thoughts and when it was in front of me it occupied my mouth. I had to trust that by letting go of obsessing I wouldn't go hungry, starve or die by not thinking about food 24/7. I had to realize *food* did not make me overweight: it was how I used it. (The amounts I ate were more than what my body needed, even though I made healthier food choices.)

When your overall meal plan is based on wholesome foods (this will be covered shortly), you will find that you eat processed foods less often, without feeling restriction. *Remember that* food *is neutral.* There are not good foods or bad foods. Some are less healthy than others and not all food should be eaten in the same quantities. When you're eating habits are healthy approximately 80% of the time, there is room to indulge or have a treat on occasion without stressing about its effect on your figure or health. Even the healthiest foods can have negative effects on your size if you are not conscious of your portions or amounts.

Nighttime Eater

Back in my corporate days, I fell into this category as well. I went for large periods of time without eating because I was too busy or didn't have time, and then I would eat uncontrollably once I finally had the chance. I would sometimes "save" my calories until evening if I knew I was entertaining clients over dinner or if I had an evening social event (these always incorporated food).

Most of the time I ate out of hunger *and* mental exhaustion. Ironically, as an active mom I often catch myself in these same situations. On my days off from personal training, I usually get up early to get things done. I go from one task to the next, trying to get everything in before my kids wake from their naps or before it's time for carpooling pick up. Sometimes the day is nearly gone before I realize I haven't eaten for an extended period of time.

If you've been a typical diet-minded person, you may tend to eat this way as well. You eat very little during the day—feeling like you're "doing so well"—then assume your willpower can carry you through the entire evening. The truth is, severely restricting your calories for a long period of time can be a formula for overeating. Many nighttime eaters eat more calories in the evening compared to what they would eat if they spread out their food consumption during the day.

It's important for you to begin each day by eating breakfast. People who eat breakfast tend to consume fewer calories overall compared to non-breakfast eaters. And when I say breakfast, I mean more than a cup of coffee or a can of Diet Coke!

Some people think snacking is a bad thing. They try not to snack between meals and feel proud when they can make it to their next big meal without eating in between. Realize that snacking throughout the day can be a good thing, especially if you're eating healthier foods.

For this eating type, it's better to eat small amounts when you can, rather than starve all day and binge later. You need to make a conscious effort to have healthy snacks or meals with you during the day if stopping to eat is difficult. By making an effort to eat small amounts during the day, you will have more energy and most likely be more effective at your duties. In addition, you'll avoid hitting starvation mode by early evening.

By spreading out your calories this way, the urge to binge in the evening can disappear. The key to avoid binges is to not let yourself get hungry. By the time you're hungry, it's already difficult to control the quantity of food you want to eat. If you can have a piece of fruit or munch on veggies, or whole wheat/grain products throughout the day, you can avoid extreme hunger. It takes mere minutes to eat a banana, an apple, a whole wheat roll, or to open a baggie of carrots or sugar snap peas. Have food with you and make time to eat it if you are constantly on the go. No matter what you do all day, you can find the time to munch on something. Raw fruits and vegetables can be consumed quickly and they take no preparation time.

Try curbing your appetite once you get home by warming up a bowl of healthy vegetable soup (see my *Boot Camp Food Manual* for recipes and menus), enjoying a piece of fruit or other low-calorie snack. Taking a minute to have a low-calorie snack before preparing dinner can help tie you over while you're preparing your meal or until dinnertime. Sometimes setting up after-dinner treat strategies can squash the mindless eating and lack of portion control that earmarks nighttime eaters.

Decide you will only eat fruits and vegetables after dinner or only take one serving of something with you (not the entire box or bag) as you sit down to eat. Eat only at the table or in the kitchen without multi-tasking. This may cut down on your volume if you are wanting to get to your favorite TV show, read, or attend to any other task. Avoid eating in front of the TV or while doing any other thing for that matter. You'll become more conscious of what and how much you eat.

"As Much as Possible before Monday Morning" Eater

Stop the dieting already! Change your mentality. NO more diets, just a healthier way of life. Dieting will ultimately make you heavier and unhealthier. Diets fail you, not your willpower or your intentions. The diets you keep trying are unrealistic and demoralizing. They drive you to "stinkin' thinkin'" by leading you to believe you're a failure. You blame yourself for not having any willpower.

By eating more balanced with vegetables, fruits, and whole grains, you will not need to deprive yourself of every treat you love, leaving you susceptible to bingeing. You will be able to enjoy your favorite treat on occasion and you will not be starving your body by taking in too few calories. The tendency to overindulge means you being too restrictive by not allowing yourself small indulgences or pleasures. Or when you do allow them, you may over-react to the situation by thinking this is the last time you will ever eat that food again and binge. Know that when you've dieted, it's the *method* that's been messing up, not you!

You need to consciously create a nutrition plan to know which types of foods should be eaten in abundance and which foods should be eaten sparingly. Eat your favorite foods in appropriate portions. (We will cover this in the Meals section.) If you are allowed anything you desire in moderation, you will be able to beat the urge to overeat it on a regular basis.

Rather than go for a long period of time before you start eating healthy again, get through your splurge meal, then get back on track with your next snack or meal. Don't wait until the weekend is over to correct a bad meal choice or unhealthy eating habit. Do it at the next meal. Do it now!

Emotional Eater

I've learned that some bodies are just not willing to be deprived or subjected to punishment and restriction (no matter how bad you want to starve yourself or lose weight). Most of these bodies are the one's carrying around extra weight as a substitute to feeling hugged, warmth, accepted or secure. Emotional eating is easy and requires little effort.

Food is readily available and provides immediate effects. Eating feels good and we know the response we'll get from it. As a society, we have an obsession with thinness and dieting heightens our preoccupation with food. A wise but anonymous person once said, "Chocolate is cheaper than therapy and you don't need an appointment."

Internal messages create your emotional state. Your perception can make you feel stressed, anxious, worried, or depressed and you'll be more likely to binge or overeat.[6] If you find yourself continually using food when you are happy, angry, sad, frustrated, bored, lonely, stressed or disappointed, then most likely you are not listening to your true hunger or satiety. Emotions are the key player for you and you must learn to master them. Don't allow emotions to dictate your actions or your results. Be active, and take control of your emotions. By taking responsibility of your emotions, you can choose to act rather than react with food.

Rather than turning to food to medicate your emotional needs, write down a list of replacement ideas to try. When an emotion is triggered and you find yourself going to the pantry, try calling a friend, cleaning a room or a drawer, reading a book, surfing the Internet, going on a walk, riding a bike, doing something nice for someone else, or going to the gym. Sometimes we tend to overreact to things that don't have to be so huge. We make them huge by the way we respond.

Before you react, evaluate how monumental the issue really needs to be. Find a few activities that you could do rather than eat. Begin paying closer attention to your actions. Sometimes emotional eaters will fill their downtime, loneliness, or boredom with mindless eating. If that's the case for you, find a distraction that will give you something to do or a way to feel better. After all, we truly know that eating in response to these situations only sets us up for more disappointment and frustration.

---

6   *Phil pg. 51*

BodyJoy Tip

When should you see a trainer or other specialist?

Sometimes a good, responsible nutrition or workout book can keep you on track. But then there are times when working on your physique, counting calories, exercising and stress management are just too overwhelming. When you feel emotionally or mentally overwhelmed it is good to seek professional guidance. Consider a dietician, certified personal trainer, or psychologist. Dieticians and certified personal trainers who keep current with industry trends as well as psychologists all work with people's thoughts and feelings as they relate to food in addition to counting calories and analyzing food logs. You can utilize these services long-term or until you feel like you can handle everything on your own.

I've dealt with emotional eating in a number of my clientele and I've used food to cope with issues and feelings myself. I'm an emotionally fueled person. The stimulus may be different for each of us. I've seen individuals use food to cope with events ranging from expectations and pressures of not feeling good enough or of childhood neglect, to mental, physical and sexual abuse and other serious traumas. Some of my clients began to thrive after seeing a therapist to resolve their emotional issues. Others have found alternatives other than food to deal with their problems.

What makes you happy? What gives you an endorphin rush or that "runner's high"? Is it physical movement? Is it relationships? Recognize the small things in life and appreciate them. Be grateful for the little things.

I found that using a food log and recording *why* I ate, not only when I ate, was helpful in recognizing patterns as to how I used food. This tool is successful for a number of people working on physical goals. You can read more about food logs in the *Successful Goal Setting* Chapter or you can find out more information at *www.mindybuxton.com*.

The most important thing for an emotional eater to do is to identify *why* you are eating. Before you eat something, ask yourself, "Am I really hungry?" or "Do I really want that?" If the answer is NO—put the food away and get what you really need—a drink, a minute to relax, release from your stress, or do something that will make yourself happy. You can also ask yourself, "What does eating do for me?" Is it fulfilling an emotional need? Try getting to the bottom of why you have that emotion.

Perhaps if you resolve the problem, you will be less inclined to eat. Often this is something that cannot be addressed on your own, and that's all right. It may require seeing a therapist, talking to your doctor, a family member or friend or going to a nutritionist or certified trainer to resolve issues. It's okay to ask for help. We all need help at some time or another! (This is how I found my trainer, and he played a huge roll in helping me improve my body and life.)

The important thing is that you take whatever action is necessary to address these issues so you can progress with your goals. There is no way out of this cycle except through addressing your feelings and finding a balance between your reason and your emotions. This type of eating affects you both mentally and physically, so it's vital to get these issues addressed and resolved. Your size, health and happiness depend on it!

On-the-Run Eater

If you find yourself on the go, remember there are healthy solutions to getting food fast rather than picking up fast-food. If your schedule is so overbooked that you are constantly on the go, make sure your food choices are healthy ones. Fresh vegetables, fruits, and nuts are just as easy to grab as a candy bar or other processed treat. If you take them with you at the start of your day, you eliminate the need to have to make an additional stop for food. Be sure to carry a water bottle with you.

It's important to stay hydrated so you don't mistake thirst for hunger pains. Take a look at how you organize your time and make time to eat (even if it's in the car or walking between appointments). It's better to eat when you can than starve yourself the entire day.

BodyJoy Tip

Smaller meals or snacks more frequently throughout the day can be the key to having energy and avoiding hunger.

If you pay attention to what you are eating, you will have fewer opportunities to mindlessly eat an entire bag of something as you are rushing around throughout the day. This is typical for on-the-run eaters. Many consume more calories munching throughout the day than if they would have sat down and eaten three square meals. If paying attention to what you eat is hard for you, separate servings of nuts, vegetables, fruit pieces, or dried fruit into snack-size baggies. This way your portions are measured out and you can't overeat unintentionally. Track your food by writing it down for a few days so you can calculate just how many servings of pretzels, chips or other convenience foods you eat while going about your day.

Run into a supermarket for lunch or a snack rather than always going to a drive through. Just make some time in your day for eating. When you are eating smaller amounts more often, it is not as disruptive to your schedule. It takes less time to grab something small every now and then than to take an entire lunch hour to eat.

I tend to eat this way the days I work at the gym. I have a different client come in each hour and rather than taking one full hour to eat lunch, I snack on fruits, vegetables, half a sandwich, and nuts in between my appointments. I especially think sugar snap peas, grape tomatoes, blueberries, pears, apples, and trail mix are convenient options.

I try not to go more than three hours without having something to eat. This keeps my energy level where I need it and I can keep hunger at bay. I always carry a water bottle around with me so I can drink all day long. Proper hydration aids in keeping your stomach full. By dinner, I assess how much I've eaten throughout the day and then adapt my dinner size accordingly. If you get in an adequate amount throughout the day, try having a more modest amount at night.

Strategy 9

Becoming a More Intuitive Eater

by Recreating your Mealtime Mentality

Despite which eating type(s) you fall under, we all can use some tips for becoming a more intuitive eater. First, become aware of your "mealtime mentality". Mine used to consist of eating my food on my feet, in front of the fridge, pantry or while preparing meals. I would scarf my food down and be on my way the second I was done. I ate in front of the television, reading, or at my computer regularly.

I found I ate much of my food mindlessly, without really tasting it or enjoying it. Most of the time, I didn't notice I was even eating until I consumed more than I actually needed. Assess what your current mealtime mentality is. Whatever that may look like, here are some helpful suggestions. Take what will work for you to improve your own mealtime mentality.

Keep your meals at the table or counter this will provide a designated spot to eat where you can focus or concentrate on the task at hand—eating. When it's time to eat, avoid multi-tasking. When possible avoid eating on-the-go, in front of the television or at your desk or computer. Sit down to eat your food. Avoid eating your food while you are standing and preparing it or munch on veggies if you're starving. Discover which foods you truly enjoy and incorporate them into more meals or snacks.

Assess which foods you eat mindlessly or eat without experiencing pleasure and consume them less—if at all. You can do this by analyzing your food logs and noticing what you ate, how much you ate, and how you felt. Which foods are your vices? Find a better way to eat them and treat yourself to them on occasion. With your food logs, notice your rituals or habits. Do you always have chips or fries with sandwiches? Notice when you are eating processed or fast foods and decide if you need them on a daily basis. Could you get by on three days a week or once a week? Could you substitute fruit or vegetables for the processed foods at some meals? Pay attention to what you're eating on a regular basis.

Eating can be a pleasurable experience on several levels. When you eat, do you enjoy every aspect of your meal? Are you aware of flavors, aromas, textures and feelings? Can you appreciate the feeling and experience of eating? Eating can be a nourishing, wonderful experience. You should be able to enjoy your meals. Treat them as indulgences. Know that you can feel indulged without engorging yourself. Taking in all aspects that your meal has to offer can intensify and create a more gratifying experience.

Is your food high quality? Smaller amounts of higher-quality foods can provide richer, more satisfying flavor. Choose quality over quantity. Flavorful cheeses, fine chocolates and fresh vegetables and fruits are just a few examples. Chew your food slowly and savor each bite. (This is still a hard one for me.)

When eating with others, enjoy the company, learn about each other's day and connect. I love having meals at the table; however, my husband still lobbies to eat in front of the TV when he can. Even if it's just lunch at home with my daughters, I push for meals at the table. I hope to instill this important concept in them so they can avoid the mindless consumption that packed unnecessary pounds onto my childhood frame. As a child and teenager, I ate huge amounts in front of TV, but I hated how I looked because of it!

I enjoy "table-time" to visit with my girls and learn about their thoughts and ideas. With the fast-pace world of today it seems you have to purposely make time to sit down and talk to others. What better way to do it than over a meal? Dinner is our time of the day as a family to sit down, unwind, refuel our bodies and enjoy spending time together free from distractions. Some of my favorite moments with my daughters have been around the dinner table. This is where they will grow up eating.

How much of your food is prepared yourself? The more you prepare, the more you are aware of what goes into your meals. An intuitive eater takes charge. They are masters of their pleasures as well as their restraints. If you choose to enjoy a larger serving at lunch, compensate by eating a little less at dinner. If you choose to have a few pieces of bread out of the breadbasket with your meal, maybe skip the dessert or vice versa. Intuitive eaters pick their moments and know when to compensate so everything balances out.

Finally, assess your daily experiences. Your purpose is to be happy, thrive and experience joy. Make sure your day is full of several simple pleasures. Appreciation will allow you to create the best experience possible. Be mindful of the small things; maybe they are your home, clothing, family, friends, careers, neighborhoods, the sunshine, snow, a minute for yourself, the ability to move, etc. These are all things we can take for granted.

Find joy and pleasure in your day and show appreciation for your life and those things that can bring it meaning. Use part of your workout time to think of things to be grateful for. This simple but important concept can have a huge impact on your perception, body image, eating habits and movement. Let gratitude and appreciation help you create a better experience with your body and your life.

List 5 ways you can improve your eating behavior:

1. _____

2. _____

3. _____

4. _____

5. _____

Strategy 10

Participate in "The Ultimate Dining Experience"

The next meal you enjoy out, no matter where you end up eating, I want you to participate in the "Ultimate Dinning Experience". If you've never experienced this before, you're in for a treat! It goes like this:

Preparation

Throughout the day, anticipate your meal out. Hopefully you are going to a favorite restaurant or out to a new place you've been dying to try. Make sure you go to your meal at a content hunger level. You aren't full of course, but you're definitely not starving.

At the meal

Arrive at the restaurant or at the dinner table feeling content, because you're not starving. Once you're seated take a look around. Notice what you see. Notice what you smell. Notice how your surroundings make you feel. Take in the atmosphere. Observe all it has to offer. Your surroundings, your company and your mood or feelings are all part of the dinning experience. So often we place the emphasis solely on the food.

Start drinking your water and look over the menu. If you've been served a starter, like bread or chips, wait until you've ordered to begin eating it. Order anything you feel like having. Yes, you heard me right. Your trainer is encouraging you to go with whatever you feel like having. Don't judge your pick. Don't worry about calories, fat or proteins. Order your meal of choice without feeling guilty.

As you eat, whether it's the starter or your entrée, I want you to TASTE each and every bite. This means putting your mind into what you're doing and maybe eating a little slower than usual. It's common for us to eat without tasting our food. Think about that for a minute. Most of the time we are squeezing our meals in between other important appointments or grabbing a bite to eat on the run while we're focused on driving, talking on the phone or a number of other duties we are in need of accomplishing.

For this meal, pay attention to each bite. Notice how it tastes, how it smells, and how it feels in your mouth. Notice the feelings you get from it. Explore the flavors or seasonings and textures. Be present in the moment and experience the joy food can bring you. Studies have shown that we really enjoy the first few bites of something, then we habitually do "hand to mouth" activity mindlessly, either because the food's in front of us or we're preoccupied and don't notice the lack of joy or satisfaction.

Once you're pleasure level sinks lower with that food item, move on to the next and repeat your exercise. If your experience is like mine, you'll realize you don't have to eat too much of something, if you're mindfully eating to enjoy it then be ready for something else. You may also notice if you really stop when the pleasure sensation is gone, you don't eat a huge amount of any one thing. Eating takes a little longer and you won't end up uncomfortably stuffed. When you're present in the moment, you may find you don't enjoy eating something just because it's in front of you. It's easier to put the fork down when you stop experiencing satisfaction.

Mindful eating can help decrease extra large portions or eating food for the sake of just doing something even if you're not hungry. When you're paying attention you can shift away from food onto something you really need if you know what you're feeling. Food should and can be a pleasurable experience if you're experiencing it appropriately.

Strategy 11

Successful Goal Setting

"Success is the sum of small efforts, repeated day in and day out."

—Robert Collier

Losing body fat and inches is not a matter of willpower; it's a matter of awareness, preparation and planning! By identifying why you eat, having the right perception and learning proper goal-setting techniques, you have the power to change your physique. Setting goals reminds me of New Year's resolutions.

How many Januarys have you set goals regarding your health, weight, and fitness? Do you find yourself setting the same goals every year since you have not yet achieved them? While many people resolve to change their behavior every January—lose body fat, eat healthy, get in shape, and exercise more—the sad truth is that by mid-February most of their good intentions have fallen by the wayside. Part of the problem may be that they haven't properly learned how to set goals.

Goals are essential to exercise consistency and weight-loss adherence. If you have a clearly defined purpose when designing your goals, you are much more likely to continue—and even to look forward to your workouts and healthy meals. Of course, all of us have moments when we simply don't feel like putting in the effort. Illness, family demands, work issues and other crises can set back our efforts for days or even weeks. However, if you have well-defined goals that are important to you, you will be more inclined to resume your healthy routine quickly.

A goal must be both quantifiable and attainable. If these criteria aren't met, the goal is nonspecific and not meaningful. Nonspecific goals cannot be achieved and are likely to result in frustration. In order for a goal to be quantifiable, it must have measurable parameters. For example, losing 20 pounds in three months is a quantifiable goal.

Other examples of quantifiable goals include reducing your waistline by three inches in one month or dropping one dress size in six weeks. Conversely, "wanting to look good" is not a quantifiable goal. This is subjective and cannot be measured by defined standards. In fact, such a goal is doomed to lead to disappointment and frustration. When it comes to setting successful goals, you must outline specifics.

In order for a goal to be attainable, it must be realistic. For example, losing 20 pounds in three months is a realistic and attainable goal. Losing a dress or pant size in two months is realistic and attainable. Losing 90 pounds or three sizes in one month is not. If a goal is not attainable, it can make your endeavors feel pointless. It is better to set modest goals that are within reach. This enables greater success with your overall objective.

Manageable Steps & Short-Term Goals

Simply deciding to reshape your body isn't enough. You need to create a strategy. Once you decide what you want to accomplish, you need to map out in great detail how you're actually going to do it. Will you cut down on desserts? Will you exercise four mornings a week? Are you going to lift weights at the gym on Tuesday and Thursday nights?

Once you have formulated your overall goal, break it down into short time frames. Use a time frame of no more than three months.

This is a reasonable period of time in which to see noticeable results without feeling like the goal is taking an eternity to achieve. For example, losing 25 pounds might appear to be a daunting task, but losing two pounds a week for three months doesn't sound so overwhelming. Keep in mind it's safe to lose one to two pounds a week. More than this per week results in water and muscle loss—not body fat.

It's also important to determine how you'll handle obstacles. Be sure to determine likely obstacles based on which type of eater you are. (See Strategies 5 and 6.) If you travel frequently for work, you might tuck exercise bands or other workout gear in your suitcase and try to stay at hotels with workout facilities.

If you tend to eat when you are anxious (or otherwise emotionally triggered), make a list of activities you can do instead. Remember, you need a plan! Don't think you'll just deal with temptation as it comes up. Unfortunately, you can't just wing it when it comes to ingrained habits. If it were that easy to change them, all of us would be at our best bodies all the time!

While long-term goals are valuable, be sure to make short-term goals as well. By focusing on these smaller benchmarks, you'll stay mindful of what you're doing and increase your chances of success. It's important to have a big-picture goal, but it's the significant short-term goals that get you to the end result. It's all about small changes or baby steps to see long-term results and success.

Let me tell you about my client Brent. A few years ago, Brent came to me for marathon training. He had a difficult time running his first race. He ran it unconditioned and as a result he experienced several injuries that affected him for months after his marathon. His long-term goal was to improve his physical condition to avoid getting injured during his next marathon.

After setting his long-term goal, he couldn't just expect to show up at the start line and run the marathon of his life. We had to create manageable steps and establish smaller, short-term goals, which included assessing his posture to pick exercises to improve his alignment, setting a specific amount of cardio activity during each week, going on a long run each week, gradually increasing his mileage on his long runs, following the walk-run theory, designing a stretching program for after each run, and creating a nutrition plan to fuel his body for the activity he was performing.

We took his twenty-four week program one week at a time. Brent was the first marathon runner I had trained. The day he approached me, I thought running 26.2 miles sounded overwhelming. But halfway through Brent's training I realized I was conditioning myself right along with him to prepare for this marathon. After all, I couldn't just drive next to him in the car while he ran his long runs. (Though some days I wished I could!)

Running a marathon was something I never thought about doing—ever. By the last week of Brent's race training—after accomplishing all of the short-term goals and following his outlined program—we were both ready for his marathon. Not only did Brent and I complete the marathon, but he improved his time by nearly forty minutes and that night he was walking around uninjured and able to celebrate. Brent and I both experienced firsthand how manageable steps or short-term goals can lead to successful outcomes.

Incentives and Recognition

Whenever possible, create incentives to help you reach your goals. Having positive rewards on a regular basis can encourage you and help you stay motivated to reach your ultimate goal. It's important to reward yourself for reaching your smaller or short-term goals. Think how good it feels when you get a compliment from a friend or co-worker when they notice you've lost a few pounds.

I know I always feel more motivated to keep working on my goals when others acknowledge my results. But don't just rely on those around you for positive feedback. Provide it for yourself. Encourage yourself by providing your own "pats on the back" and recognition (try out your positive self-talk!) when you accomplish each manageable step.

Use non-food-based rewards to provide encouragement and the determination to keep you motivated. (This is particularly important for emotional eating types.) An incentive can be something as simple as standing in front of the mirror and telling yourself how great you are looking or something more elaborate like a trip or weekend getaway. You could buy new workout gear or treat yourself to a post-workout massage or a session with a personal trainer. If you want to lose sizes, buy an expensive pair of jeans that's your goal size. The thought of having a pair of pants sitting unused in your closet may be an effective motivator to get you to workout and eat healthier.

Some of my clients treat themselves to a new book, a pedicure or manicure, a facial, new make-up or a piece of new workout equipment as recognition for reaching their short-term goals. The more recognition you provide, the more support and encouragement you will have along the road to success. Let recognition and incentives be driving forces fueling you toward your ultimate goal. What are some incentives that will work for you?

_____

_____

_____

_____

_____

Accountability

Create accountability by having to report your progress to another individual. Getting others involved in your fitness efforts will provide a support network that can spur you on to greater heights.[7] Use accountability to your advantage: it doesn't need to be a punishment or a negative thing. It doesn't need to be "big brother" watching over you. It's a tool to keep you focused and provide the support you deserve while you are making changes to your lifestyle and creating new and better habits.

This is one of my largest roles as a personal trainer. I'm the person to whom my clients report and come to on a regular basis for support, encouragement and direction. Several of the clients I train have been with me for over six years and many have used trainers for over ten years. They know what to do in the gym. They understand how hard they need to work out to see results. So why do they continue to personal train? They need accountability in order to reach their goals. Some of them will take breaks or go months at a time on their own, but as soon as they see their results stop, they return to training.

Accountability is essential for many of us to reach our goals. Most of us cannot provide it for ourselves. I set up consultation times during each year to meet with my trainer to measure, assess my body fat percentage and discuss my goals. Whenever I feel my efforts are not producing results, I immediately arrange an appointment. Good trainers practice what they preach by applying the same principles in keeping their own bodies on track and reaching their desired results.

---

[7] *Schoenfield, Brad CPFT, CSCS, AFAA trainer and author of best-selling Sculpting Her Body Perfect and Look Great Naked.*

Don't get discouraged if you need to report to another individual. It's not sign of weakness; it's a smart step to take to ensure you see results! Whether you choose a personal trainer, workout partner, spouse or a friend, tell someone about your goal and establish follow-up times with that person. Some people need to meet on a weekly, monthly, or quarterly basis. This number should correlate to where you are in terms of accomplishing your goals. We all have easier moments and more difficult ones to work through.

BodyJoy Tip

Keeping an exercise and food log is one of the most beneficial tools for keeping you on track toward your health and fitness goals.

Set up your accountability meetings according to how often you need feedback and support. Some times you may go longer periods without checking in and other times you may need to meet weekly. These follow-up visits can help get you back on track before you get too frustrated or they can serve as additional encouragement to keep your forward momentum. You will find being accountable to another person will provide tremendous support, encouragement and reinforcement to keep you on the right track to success.

Use my website *www.mindybuxton.com* as an accountability and support resource. Log on to find online support from personal trainers, helpful information and tips. Use it to record your daily logs or to find recommended exercise products. Resources such as these are available to you. Use them regularly so your goals can be achieved. I have also included a list of recommended resources at the end of my book. Do what it takes for you to see results and achieve body joy.

Tracking Progress

An exercise and food log allows you to record workouts and nutrition information such as what you eat, how much you eat, when you eat, and why you eat. By doing this, you can identify habits and understand when you need to replace coping methods of eating with other activities such as exercising, calling a friend, reading, or browsing the Web. The majority of individuals who have reached success with their physical goals recorded their nutrition and exercise as they tracked their goals. These tools allow you to monitor your progress.

By recording what you eat, you can become aware of which areas need improvement and which are on track with your goals. Tracking your food consumption doesn't need to be a full-time job.

You won't need to log every bite you consume for the rest of your life. Keep the log for a couple weeks to figure out your eating patterns. If there's only one time of day that is difficult for you, just record that time. Make notes in your planner, e-mail yourself or leave yourself phone messages to help you jot down your information at the end of the day. If it is easier for you, record each meal as you eat it.

A food and exercise log can be maintained on a simple piece of paper, in a notebook, or on a computer. There are online resources which calculate your caloric intake so you do not have to look up calories or macronutrients yourself. The most effective food log I have found is a web-based program that automatically adds up calories and nutrients as you enter what you've eaten.

I have clients who go from being stuck at plateaus to losing one pound each week once they begin logging their food online. I used this program to reach my personal best and was able to achieve my lowest weight and body fat percentage. I finally created the body I always wanted and I maintain it by logging my food daily online. You can visit *www.mindybuxton. com* for more details about web-based food logs.

In this book you will find Daily Log Sheets you can use to begin recording your food and activity. You can also do this online. Keeping a log will teach you how to analyze yourself. You can share it with the person you are accountable to, your trainer or dietician, or keep it for your own private information. This process provides assistance in learning how you can improve your activity and eating in order to achieve your goal.

For many of my clients, tracking information is the key to getting them going again when they hit a rut. They may think they have an idea of how they are eating, but once they actually see it on paper they realize they may have underestimated the calories they consumed or overestimated how many calories they actually burn. Tracking information for your fat-loss goals and health improvement can be as important as balancing your checkbook—it keeps you aware of what you can afford when it comes to calories.

Attitude Check: Are you remaining positive?

Simply setting goals will not ensure long-term success. Your attitude, outlook and self-talk must reflect your ability to succeed. It seems difficult to regularly exercise when you detest working out. If you view exercise solely as a vehicle to get you down the road to your goal, you're setting yourself up for failure. It's important to develop the mental and emotional skills you need to actually enjoy being active.

Have you ever focused on what you would like to gain from your goals? Most of the time, we tend concentrate only on what we would like to lose or what we need to stop or cut out. Focus on what you can gain from the changes you will make in order to achieve your goals. You could gain more energy, a healthier lifestyle, less sickness, less stress better, move easier, look better, or even receive pleasure from moving and exercising. The process of changing your body does not need to be a punishment. There are many options of activities out there, find something you can enjoy doing.

When you can enjoy exercise for its own sake, you become intrinsically motivated—motivated from the inside out. How do you develop intrinsic motivation? Select physical activities that you enjoy to create a positive experience. Sign up for a kickboxing class, use an exercise video, go for a run or join friends for a long walk each day. Whatever makes you *feel good* is what will work.

If you have never been able to enjoy it, you may not have found the right exercise yet. Keep trying new activities until you find one you can accept. Activity should be about the experience, not just the end result. Pay attention to the immediate benefits: improved energy, stress relief, and the adrenaline surge while you're moving. You'll be amazed at how much more enjoyable exercise can be when you're not dreading just "another boring workout." There is some type of exercise out there for you.

Associate yourself with people who are active, healthy and support your goals of looking and feeling better. These people can provide an additional positive support and make lifestyle transitions easier. I assist in Fitness Challenges on a regular basis. It's amazing to watch how much better the individuals who "band together" to meet each other for workouts do, in comparison to the individuals who don't participate in group classes or partner workouts. They're not as motivated to keep exercising on a regular basis and they even see fewer results in inches and body fat loss.

Remember to work on improving your self-respect and body image as you are accomplishing your goals. A person who is happy with him or herself can be happier with other people as well. A positive outlook and attitude can make all the difference in the world regarding your success. Attitude can be the deciding factor in whether you will reach your goal or if you will fail. If you know you can do it, you will! Stay positive! The old adage still rings true, you can do anything you put your mind to.

Identify Obstacles

You may call them excuses, reasons, or obstacles—it really doesn't matter. Determine what's stopping you from achieving your fitness goals. Be a person who learns from trial and success, not trial and failure. Identify what has hindered your success in the past, incorporate overcoming your obstacles in your new goal-setting process, and, this time, *expect* to see results.

Common Obstacles: Time, Lack of Planning, and Support

If **time** is your obstacle, look for ways to build fitness activities into your daily life—walk the stairs at lunchtime or circle the field during your child's soccer game. Begin getting up a half hour earlier each day to exercise. Don't commit to a program you can't maintain. If you miss a day or two, don't abandon exercise altogether. Simply pick up where you left off and begin moving again. If you suffer from a **lack of planning**, schedule workouts on your calendar and stick to your program. Once you've molded being active into a habit, it will become second nature to you.

If you are lacking **support**, talk to your spouse or partner and let him or her know how important your workouts are to your overall well-being. Explain to your kids how important being active is, and then search for activities your family can enjoy together. You will probably see that they completely understand how important this is to you and they can be great motivators if you need their help.

Change may not be easy, but it's possible with the right keys to successful goal setting. Remember, it isn't the act of setting a goal or starting a new habit that counts, it's keeping with them that's important. Repetition in thinking and in doing creates new habits; a healthier life-style will eventually be as automatic as your current one.

Expect that you will experience times that are more difficult or scheduling conflicts along the way. We all face these issues and we all have setbacks no matter what we are trying to achieve. They are part of the process. Rather than getting frustrated or giving up, endure through these times and remain focused on your ultimate goal.

> *"Never in your life will you be without emotional pain and stress, problems, challenges and difficult moments are simply a part of living. You know that if things are going well at work, for example, you can count on conflict at home, or vice versa. There is rarely a time in your life when all is at peace and balance. That's neither good nor bad; it is simply the ebb and flow of how life works. To be alive means to experience emotions, painful or otherwise."*

> —Dr. Phil McGraw

The BodyJoy Formula to Successful Goal Setting

- ✓ Determine your overall goals.
- ✓ Define how you will achieve your goals in terms of specific behaviors.
- ✓ Assign a timeline to your goals.
- ✓ Break down your goals into manageable steps.
- ✓ Create accountability.
- ✓ Identify obstacles.

Use the following sheet to record your goals and assign a timeline to when you would like to achieve them. Create accountability and establish your commitment. No one can change your body for you—only you have the power to create change within yourself. Don't wait to begin working on your goals until it's convenient or until things have calmed down. That's the formula for failing to achieve nothing.

I have never understood the following comments:

> *"I will go to the gym once I lose weight!" or "I will get a trainer once I am in better shape."*

Instead, use these measures as a means to achieving your goals. A gym is a place where you can lose weight and a trainer can help you get in better shape. Search for a gym you feel comfortable at. They're out there!

Sometimes a trainer can ease the stress of being at a gym and not knowing what to do. Stop finding excuses and do what is necessary to progress. Set your goals right now and begin working on your best body today! Besides, you never know what great new friends you might meet at the gym and you will be surprised at how you may even long to go to the gym or not feel quite right when you haven't made the time to go.

BodyJoy Steps to Success

Make a commitment. What are you willing to do or what will it take for you to see results?

Make your goal a priority every single day. Assess and plan out time during your week to work on your goal.

- Be consistent to create new habits.
- Endure through plateaus/setbacks. Expect to have them and don't equate minor setbacks with failure. They are part of the process!
- Evaluate your setbacks and plateaus; see if you can do anything to change or avoid them.
- Be willing to try new things and challenge yourself.
- Incorporate your goals into family or friend time.
- Know that improving yourself will allow you to better care for family and friends.
- Use exercise or movement to cope with stress, depression, or other negative emotions.

Health & Fitness Goal Sheet

Specifically, and in detail, what do you want to achieve?

What exactly will you do to achieve your goal? (List behaviors/actions you must change, stop, or begin.)

Step 1.

Step 2.

Step 3.

Step 4.

Step 5.

When you achieve your goal you want to feel: _____(i.e., more energetic, proud of your size, at peace with your body).

What is the time frame of your goal? _____ (one month, one year, fifteen weeks, etc.)

Break down your goal into manageable steps (drop a size per month, for example).

Step 1.

Step 2.

Step 3.

Identify possible obstacles and how you'll respond to those obstacles.

Who will you be accountable to? _____

(Name of person and how often you'll report)

If there were ever a time to dare to make a difference,
To embark on something worth doing,
It is now.

Not for any grand cause necessarily
But for something that tugs at your heart,
Something that's your aspiration
Something that's your goal.
You owe it to yourself to make your days here count.
Have fun. Dig deep.
Stretch. Dream Big.

Know that things worth doing seldom come easy.
There will be good days.
There will be bad days.
There will be times when you want to turn around,
Pack it up, and call it quits.
Those times tell yourself
That you are pushing yourself,
That you are not giving up.
Persist.

Because with a goal,
Determination,
And the right tools,
You can do great things.
You are worth it!
Trust.

Believe in the incredible power of the human mind.
Of doing something that makes a difference.
Of working hard.
Of seeing results.
Of making changes.
Of feeling great.
Of all the things that will cross your path.

The start of something new
Brings the hope of something great.
Anything is possible.
There is only one you.
And you will pass this way only once.
Do it now!

—Anonymous

Movement

Movement is an essential element in achieving your goal. We would all be slimmer and healthier if we focused more on activity and movement than on diet. One of the best tools for finding and maintaining your best body is movement. When you move, your body burns calories. The more you move the more calories you burn. Even the simplest activities can increase the rate of calories burned during the day. Whether doing household chores, playing with children, or taking the stairs rather than the elevator; these simple activities are key to increasing the amount of calories you burn. It's not just about your exercise, but about your overall movement on a daily basis.

Strategy 12

Move It To Lose It!

Daily Movement

The technology of our time has made it easy not to move much. We can call our friends, family and neighbors, change the channel on the television, and play electronic games all while sitting in a chair or on the couch. Even running errands or carpooling has changed with the invention of automatic car doors giving us less of a need to get out of our seats.

We have little incentive to get up and move to accomplish most of our daily tasks. Movement entails burning calories, using your muscles and joints, and it requires bending, twisting and turning. You should aim to move as much as possible during the day. This way you can improve the number of calories you burn before you even get in a workout.

Add movement to your day any way you can. Go on a walk with your spouse or kids, walk to your neighbor's house to visit, go walking with your friends, take your dog for a walk, do yard work, clean the house, take out your garbage *everyday* rather than once a week, make several trips taking in your groceries, balance on one leg while brushing your teeth, play active games with your children or grandchildren. Start a walking group. Walk to and from destinations when possible.

There are so many ways to add movement to your daily schedule. Take the stairs at work or in buildings, park in the furthest parking stall available, walk your shopping cart back to the store entrance, or clean out your car. You've got to move it to lose it! Little bits of activity add up in big ways. The more you move, the more you'll lose!

List ways you can increase your daily movement.

_____

_____

_____

_____

_____

_____

_____

_____

Exercise & Physical Activity

Nike states it best: **Just Do It!** One of our biggest problems as a nation is that we eat too much and move too little. It's as simple as that. If you find time on a regular basis to be physically active, your weight-loss goals will be achieved much faster than if you improve your nutrition alone. Eating and exercise can directly affect each other. They seem to follow the law of motion.

Have you noticed that when you work out more often, your food choices tend to be healthier? Exercise makes you feel better and when you feel better it is generally easier to eat better. Have you also noticed that that first workout seems to be the toughest? Once you've made it through the first one, it gets easier to go the next day, then the next, etc.

Set the wheels in motion and begin exercising on a regular basis. Soon you'll realize that you might need to spend a little more time in the gym to feel as though you've really worked out. This is good—it means you're getting into shape!

It's important to make exercise a priority in your life: weight management and your health depend on it. The benefits of physical activity are numerous. It helps:

- Prevent disease
- Strengthen and tone your body
- Control weight and size
- Improve self-respect
- Improve metabolism
- Increase stamina and endurance
- Enhance flexibility
- Improve sleep quality
- Manage stress
- Improve overall quality of life

BodyJoy Tip

Inactivity is as much a health risk as smoking!

The most important commitment you can make is to exercise on a regular basis. Commit to becoming more active. Require more of yourself and start moving. It doesn't matter if you're athletic or not. Not having enough time is no excuse. Sir Winston Churchill said, "Sometimes it is not good enough to do your best; you have to do what's required."

Movement is a prerequisite to seeing fat loss and a decrease in inches. No matter whom you are or what you do, you can make the effort to move on a regular basis.

BodyJoy Tip

Almost any exercise can increase your oxygen intake and improve your health.

Incorporate activity and exercise wherever you can. It's not necessary to do it all at one time; however, it is important to do it on a regular basis. Treat your workout or exercise time as you would any other important appointment. Schedule it in your day and keep your appointment!

The familiar adage, "use it or lose it," applies to the human body. If you don't practice keeping your body active and flexible, you may not have the ability or mobility to function as you age.

Strategy 13

You Are an Athlete

All stages of life require you to be in motion. No matter who you are, consider yourself an athlete. You need to train or exercise according to the activities you perform. When creating an exercise program for general health and fitness or for sport, ask yourself, "What physical demands do my leisure, work or sport require?"

Select exercises that will enhance your ability to function; not detract from it. Whether you walk, run, or compete, does your exercise program reflect every movement you need to make?

Most likely you turn, twist, balance and stretch just by simply going about your day. Don't forget to focus on these important functional aspects of your body in addition to your physique. When you reach for something, really stretch and reach for it. When you lift something, keep your abdominals pulled in toward your spine and use your legs. Use your kids and your groceries to improve your fitness level.

List the physical demands of your day. (Examples: climbing stairs, twisting back to hand baby her bottle, carrying objects, sitting or standing, chasing after the bus or metro.)

_____

_____

———————————
———————————
———————————
———————————
———————————
———————————
———————————
———————————
———————————

Learn which type of exercise you prefer. Do you enjoy team sports, individual competitive sports, individual non-competitive activities or group activities? Remember that there's something for everyone. Find which activities you enjoy and have fun making them part of your life. For each sedentary activity or hobby you enjoy, match it with an active hobby or activity.

Athletes are self-motivated and take care of their "ends of the bargains" when away from their coaches. Successful athletes work very hard on their own in order to achieve their goals. When it comes to exercising or working out, it's not an option for an athlete. It's part of each day—it's part of a lifestyle.

BodyJoy Tip

Winners are too busy to be sad, too positive to be doubtful, too optimistic to be fearful, and too determined to be defeated.

Exercise *is* their job and it's a job that they love and enjoy. You can adopt the same mindset of having workouts and movement as something you do each day, just like waking each morning, eating breakfast, or going to bed. Physical activity should just be part of your day. You will get to the point where you won't even have to think about it because it's scheduled or routine and you do it because you need to.

I can coach you on what you need to do, but you are the only one who can make yourself do it! You are the one who will create your results.

Athletes don't give up. They do experience setbacks and losses, but they understand it's simply part of the process. They learn from their mistakes and continue trying to improve their performance and themselves. Have the mindset of an athlete. Don't allow yourself to give up after having one bad day of overeating, not exercising, or not seeing a visible change.

Know you don't have to wait until the next week, next day or even the next meal to recommit to improving yourself. Have the discipline to push yourself forward, even though it would be easier to stay in your old routine. Change requires sacrifice and brings countless rewards if you are able to stick with your efforts. Sacrifice your unhealthy routines or habits for healthy, supportive ones.

Several athletes use a perception method to assist them in achieving their goals. It's called mental imagery. This is a cognitive psychological skill in which the athlete uses all his or her senses to create a mental experience of a performance. You too can use this method to achieve success.

Imagery Exercise

Using imagery, you have an opportunity to experience success. Closing your eyes, see yourself at your goal size. Picture yourself getting ready to work out, performing your workout, and feeling great after finishing your workout. See yourself in the kitchen. Imagine yourself preparing a healthy snack or a healthy meal to enjoy. Focus on how much satisfaction and enjoyment you get from eating healthy.

BodyJoy Tip

"It is not the critic who counts; not the one who points out how the strong stumbled, or where the doer of deeds could have done better. The credit belongs to those in the arena; who strive valiantly; who fail and come up short again and again; who know great enthusiasm and great devotion; who are the best know in the end the triumph of high achievement; and who, at the worse, if they fail, as least they failed while daring greatly, so that their place shall never be with those timid souls who know neither victory nor defeat."

—Theodore Roosevelt

Imagine how vigorous and happy you feel. See yourself moving and accomplishing all you do on a regular basis in your goal body. See yourself exercising each day. How active and free you feel! You are invigorated and energized. Moving is easy and pleasant. You are happy and in control of your body. You experience body joy.

BodyJoy Tip

Do the mental imagery exercise on a regular basis. This will give you time
to focus on your goal and experience what success looks and feels like.

Visualize yourself at your goal size frequently. Be as descriptive as possible on how it feels, how you look and how you are. See it, feel it, taste it, and smell it! This will help you make your goals a reality. Remember the positive self-talk sentences and repeat them to yourself often. You are conditioning yourself for your life and the success you will achieve. Know you can and will do it because you're an athlete in the game of life.

Strategy 14

Unlimited Options of Physical Activity

There are different modes of exercise and each one provides essential benefits. It is important to include these different modes of exercise in your workout regimen. These include cardiovascular endurance, cardiovascular intervals, strength, flexibility, and balance.

Cardiovascular Endurance is the stamina or energy to participate in activities for a prolonged period of time. The duration can be anywhere from 5 to 60 minutes or longer. It is unnecessary to do it all at one time. If you need to squeeze in 3 ten-minute segments or get a few minutes in between tasks or appointments—it counts! What matters is the total endurance time, not if it is done all at once. A little bit is better than none and every minute, regardless of when, where, or how you do it, counts. Modes of cardiovascular endurance include, but are not limited to:

- Running
- Walking
- Cycling
- Elliptical training/gliding
- Swimming
- Stair Climbing
- Jump Roping
- Martial Arts

- Hiking
- Team Sports
- Group Fitness Classes

Cardiovascular Intervals can be performed by any mode of exercise. Rather than maintaining a certain speed, intensity, or incline, you vary one or more aspects during an interval workout. For instance, you can walk at a set pace for five minutes then increase either your incline or your speed for 1-2 minutes, recover for 1 minute, and then resume your initial pace. This can be repeated as many times as necessary in order to achieve your time or fatigue goal.

Due to their intensity, interval workouts should be shorter than endurance activities that last anywhere from 5-45 minutes total. Intervals are an efficient way to blast calories. They increase your peak (highest exercise intensity) and recovery time as well as improving your cardiovascular power. Interval activities may be performed by in activities such as:

- Group Fitness Classes
- Cycle Classes
- Running
- Walking
- Jump Roping
- Cycling
- Elliptical training/gliding
- Swimming
- Stair Climbing
- BodyGym (see *Exercise Product Recommendations*)

For sample interval ideas refer to *www.mindybuxton.com.*

Strength training is not just for bodybuilders or professional athletes. Everyone and anyone (especially women!) can benefit from strength training. Strength training is the foundation which you can create and structure your best body. It can reshape your figure and fuel your metabolism. Muscular strength is the ability to exert force or bursts of energy. It is an important part of exercise, not only because it strengthens your muscles, but because it also strengthens and/or maintains bone density, increases muscle tone, and helps you lose fat while building lean muscle mass. Examples of strength training include, but are not limited to:

- Sit-ups
- Push-ups
- Lunges
- Squats
- Free weights
- Circuit weights
- Cable weights
- Band exercises
- BodyGym

Using proper form and correct technique is essential. Many people watch someone else in a weight room or have a friend teach them. Be sure to learn correct form from a certified professional to avoid injury. You can refer to my website to learn how to pick a qualified personal trainer. No matter whom you are or what your goals are, you should incorporate at least two days of strength training into your week.

Flexibility is the ability for muscles and joints to bend and stretch. As we age, our joints and muscles become less limber and less flexible. It is important to maintain and/or increase your flexibility and balance so you can maintain your mobility. Examples of flexibility exercises include:

- Stretching
- BodyGym
- Yoga
- Pilates
- Martial Arts

Stretching or increasing your flexibility is most effective after your body is warmed up. Add stretching to the end of each workout. Stretching will help minimize muscle soreness and keep your body functioning at its best. It is unnecessary to feel pain and strain when you stretch. Just take your body to a point of gentle tension. If you cannot relax the muscle you are stretching, you are stretching too far. Stretch straps or bands can be used to assist your stretching if you have a hard time relaxing all your muscles while stretching.

Even if you only spend 2-4 minutes each day stretching, you can see results in your range of motion within a week. No other fitness goals are noticed this quickly! In addition to stretching at the end of each workout, squeeze in stretching wherever you can. Do it while watching TV, talking on the phone or even while reading a book or magazine. Get off the couch and move to the floor to stretch.

Balance is an important function for your body. Balance exercises can build leg muscles and help prevent falling. They can help keep you independent by helping you avoid injuries that may result from falling. There is a degree of overlap between strength, flexibility and balance exercises. Thus, balance can be incorporated into your strength and flexibility exercises.

Balance exercises can include:

- Stability/Therapy balls
- Dynadisks
- Wobble boards
- BodyGym
- Walking on uneven surfaces such as the sand
- Performing activity on a single leg
- Standing rather than sitting to do an activity

If you need assistance choosing exercise equipment, refer to the *Exercise Product Recommendations* or go to *www.mindybuxton.com*.

With all exercise, start slowly and listen to your body and your doctor. You can gradually increase when you're ready. For moderate endurance exercise, simply walk a little further each time you exercise and/or gradually increase the pace of your walks as the weeks pass. For strength exercise, lift a weight that you usually lift but do it more times than normal or increase the weight used. You should always be able to speak between breaths while exercising.

It's also normal to sense effort, and maybe even discomfort, but you should never sense pain, especially in your joints. Always remember to warm up slowly and to cool down gradually. If you use a personal trainer, be sure to check their credentials and to seek nationally certified individuals. Before beginning any exercise program, see your doctor or an exercise professional for screening tests and program advice. Remember, however, that the biggest risk in exercise is not starting.[8]

---

[8]   *ACSM, Health and Fitness Information Page, Public Information Page.*

How Much Exercise Is Enough?

As a personal trainer I'm asked a lot of questions. One of the most common questions I get is, "How often and how long do I need to exercise?" The answer relates to your specific goals. It's different for everyone, based on your goal and your current level of activity. Here are my recommendations.

If **maintenance** is your goal, then spending three days per week for an hour each workout day is sufficient. It seems this is enough movement to keep from gaining unwanted body fat, but not enough to warrant any loss. I feel this is the minimum amount any of us should perform in terms of warding off diseases and maintaining general wellness.

If changing is your goal, it's difficult to see improvements in either your performance of physique when you get in fewer than four exercise days/hours per week. *In my experience, a minimum of four days a week is necessary in order to lose body fat percentages and inches.* If you include high intensity in your training, it is unnecessary to work out every single day and very important to have one or two days a week to recover. When you include high-intensity activities five to six days a week rather than seven, you will have fewer injuries, a lesser rate of burnout, and a better immune system than if you pushed your body every single day.

If you are hard on your body without allowing recovery time, it could lead to burnout or over-training syndrome. For more information on over-training syndrome, go to www.mindybuxton.com. If you work out at a more moderate to low intensity level, it's advantageous to exercise at least five days a week.[9] At this intensity you can even do it every day. Whatever your workout level is, be sure you're actively exercising more days than not.

Don't be intimidated or frustrated with the amount of exercise needed to see physical changes. If you currently don't exercise, begin with even five minutes, then move up to ten and more until you reach your designated amount. Do what you are capable of and keep adapting and adding more time.

If you don't have a full hour to dedicate to exercise, split up your time and get it in with short periods throughout the day. The important thing is that you work it into your day however you can. Remember the key is

---

[9]   *ACSM, Fit Society Page Quarterly Publication, Winter 2001*

consistency! We're all different. Some people will notice results at four days a week, whereas some of us may have to do five or six days to see a difference. Find out what works for you!

Variety is Key

By including all modes or types of exercise in your routine, and by alternating these modes, you will get better results than if you were to pick just one type. I've worked at the same Health Club for over 10 years. Weekly I see many of the same people who have been there more than 10 years now.

These people have been working out on a regular basis, doing the exact same workouts, and guess what? They look just the same—even almost 10 years later. I know that many of them are trying to see improvements and are not trying to just maintain. Part of their problem is they don't include variety in their exercise program so their bodies hit a plateau or exercise rut. They exercise, but see no change. Plateaus are frustrating. Your body adapts to activity quicker than you may realize. If you are going to put in the effort to exercise, let's make sure you are going to see results from doing it!

If you perform the same workout each time you exercise, you will have a difficult time seeing results. Your body catches on when you do the same workout over and over. It's so smart that it knows exactly where you are going to take it (even if you are sweating and breathing hard) unless you keep your body guessing by mixing things up. Here are some options on keeping your workouts varied.

Option 1: You can alter or vary the time spent exercising.

Some of your workouts could take 15 minutes, some 30 or 60 minutes, etc. One week you could work out or exercise four days, the next work out five days and continue alternating back and forth. If one of my workouts ends up being short, the next one is a long one. I alternate back and forth, depending on my schedule.

Option 2: You can pick different types of exercise

Different machines when strength training or doing cardio or even different classes or exercise videos. Do a strength day, then a cardio day.

Switch from the treadmill to a bike or elliptical trainer. Take Pilates, Step, BodyGym and Strength Training classes as you rotate your workouts—not just one type of class.

Option 3: You can change the intensity

Alter the amount of weight, the speed, and/or the incline. Don't have a set weight for leg press or any other strength exercise; do it heavier one time, then lighten up the next. Walk on an incline one workout then the next workout keep your ramp level. Increase your speed for 2 minutes, and then go back to your regular pace. Whatever you do, mix up your workout so you are never doing the same thing two days in a row, let alone each time you exercise.

Once a week I push myself to my limits with both cardio and strength training. My following workout is Yoga where I can stretch and recover from tight muscles. If I go high intensity one workout, the next one is a moderate or lighter workout. I continually and purposefully switch back and forth.

Design Your Exercise Program

I recommend having a game plan or mapping out each week so you don't have to try and think about what to do once you have time to exercise. Whether exercising is old hat or new for you, it's smart to outline four or five workouts in advance so when it's time to exercise, you'll already know what to do. Make it easy by writing it down and then following your plan.

For example, your exercise log for a week could look like this:

Option 1	Option 2	Option 3	Option 4	Option 5
30 minutes walk/run or cardio machine	Pilates Class/Video	15-45 minutes Intervals on recumbent bike (or Spin class)	Upper-body strengthening exercises and stretching	45 minutes elliptical cardio machine
Lower-body strengthening exercises		Stretching	30-minute walk	10 minutes abdominal work

As mentioned earlier, variety is key! It's important to never do the same workout two days in a row and to alternate your exercise machines as well as the classes you take or exercise videos you follow. The more variety in your workouts, the faster you will see results. Every three to four weeks, create a new weekly log to follow.

Remember, these are only guidelines. You need to find an exercise program or way of getting movement in that works for you. You are unique, so what works for your friend or spouse may not work for you. I have always had a difficult time seeing inches move in my thighs and hips. Once I began adding cycling classes into my routine, I finally noticed a change in these areas. I make sure I have a couple running days and strength-training days a week as well. These help keep my body fat percentage in a healthy category.

I do Yoga once a week to re-center myself and stretch. I include at least one Pilates class a week because Pilates helped me get my waistline back to my pre-pregnancy measurements and has improved the strength in my core or mid-section. The point is that your physical activity must be effective for *you* to see results!

No one program works for everybody! Give new types of exercise a try and notice what makes your body change. Keep alternating exercises until you start to see results. Be patient. Remember, you can't get fit in just one workout!

Create 5 workout days to implement in your exercise program. Be sure to include:

- 2 cardio endurance workouts
- 1 interval cardio workout
- 2-3 strength-training workouts
- 1 flexibility and balance workout

Aim for a minimum of 30 minutes of exercise each day.

Remember, if your goal is to maintain your physique, three days or hours of exercise a week will do. If you have high-intensity workouts in your week, stick with five or six days of exercise. If your exercise intensity is more moderate to low, try getting in six or seven days a week.

Commit now: **How many days a week will you exercise?** _____

Keep adding variety to your program every three to four weeks to avoid plateaus. You can change either the duration or the time you go, the modes of exercise you perform, your speed or your incline. If you have a difficult time seeing results, refer to my website for additional assistance, *www.mindybuxton.com.* A certified personal trainer can create a personal workout program to achieve the goals you have set.

Sometimes small modifications and corrections in form or exercise activities can make major differences in the results you desire. A trainer can ensure you are doing the movements correctly so you are working every muscle you should. If your form is incorrect, not only are you setting yourself up for injury, but you won't see results the way you could if you were doing a movement correctly. This is why some people can't get their lower abdominals flat or see their hips decrease in size. Form affects your results more than you may think.

No matter if you put in 10 minutes or an hour, give yourself credit for being active. Any time is better than no time. Even on the most hectic days, put aside some time to focus on yourself and your body. Activity needs to be part of your daily schedule. Find a way to work it in!

Strategy 15

Simple Solutions to Busting Out
of Exercise Ruts or Plateaus

Low motivation or lost drive to exercise

When you lose your drive to exercise, recruit a workout buddy or a personal trainer. Having an appointment or a partner waiting can help give you that push you may need to get in your workout.

Need an extra push

When you feel comfortable in your workout or exercise program, it is time for a little push. If you do the same exercises over and over again your body has a hard time showing change. Your body may be used to your intensity level. See a personal trainer to increase your intensity or to give you options for adding variety to your program. Recruit a workout partner. Start going to group fitness classes, or try new and different classes often. Train for a specific event like a running race or bike trip.

A common finding is that individuals will put in the time, but sometimes they don't push themselves as hard as they could. Think about this; if you're going to put in the effort, make the most of your time so you can see results. Push yourself to a challenging level of intensity, wherever that limit may be for you.

Working out too intensely

Sometimes your body may need to recover a bit if you are pushing it too intensely. Try switching some of your high intense workouts to less intense, but very productive workouts like NIA, Yoga and Pilates. Some people get into the mindset that all workouts need to be painful. Don't underestimate the results you get from different modes of exercise.

Too little time

Let's face it; rarely do we have extra time. You have to *find* time to do exercise and workout. Whatever your schedule is, fit in movement where you can. Do it before your day begins, during lunch, or after the day is over. Do it at ten-minute bouts whenever it is convenient. Don't feel it has to be one whole uninterrupted hour at the gym. Be creative and fit it in where and when you can. Use your office space, home stairs or outdoors to the best of your ability.

Depression

Depression is a strong emotion that can sabotage health and fitness goals. Use exercise to help cope with your feelings. When you aren't in the mood to exercise, concentrate on the benefits you'll receive if you just get up and do it. Even if you don't want to workout or move, make yourself do it anyway. You can experience immediate benefits such as feeling an endorphin surge, getting rid of stress and tension and having a sense of accomplishment once you finish your workout. Exercise raises your serotonin levels, which can help you feel happier.

Keep in mind one mode of exercise is not better than any other. They are all important and your body needs the variety. Most people, who begin exercising and are trying to lose unwanted body fat, typically gravitate toward cardio exercise. These are individuals who do not understand that by increasing their muscle mass through strength training they will burn more calories at rest. It is important to have the benefits of cardiovascular and strength training, in addition to flexibility and interval workouts. The more variety in your program, the quicker you will see results.

Begin exercising as simply and easy as you need to—just begin! If 30 to 60 minutes a day sounds overwhelming, start by exercising only a few minutes, and then progressively increase your time. Just do it regularly. Make exercise doable, but not difficult. Start by walking, then progress to a brisk walk, and when or if you are ready, you can try running. If this is not appealing, ride a bike, swim, or doing whatever activity you can or like. Any mode of exercise will work.

Don't forget your daily physical demands. Focus on training in all planes your body must move. In your exercise program, include basic movement patterns like bending over, twisting to reach for something, or stretching up to put something away. Think back to your list containing the motions your body performs and use exercises that mimic those requirements in structuring your workouts.

List exercise activities that you enjoy or would like to try (as many as you can think of):

_____

_____

_____

_____

_____

_____

Strategy 16

Create a More Active Lifestyle

There are many ways to create a more active lifestyle, even when you don't think you can.

Turn Off the Television

The average American watches 10 hours of television per week. Use this time more effectively and if you can't turn off the tube, at least work out while you watch. You could stretch, use hand weights, or do lunges or squats during the news or your favorite program. I had one client who did abdominal work during commercials of her favorite TV show.

Hang Up the Telephone

Studies show that the average American spends 3 hours per week talking on the telephone outside of work. Instead of talking to your friends on the phone, get together and walk while you talk. I train a gentleman who's in a leadership position in his church.

Rather than having lengthy meetings in the evenings, he and his assistant go on early morning walks to take care of what details they can so their evening meetings don't last so long. They get in some exercise while saving time later in the day! Many of my neighbors meet for an exercise class or walk together. They talk while they are moving. I'm able to get in a few more miles each week by walking to a girlfriend's house in my neighborhood rather than driving.

Get Organized

Being organized can free between 1 and 10 hours each week. Keep your workout gear handy and schedule time to work out just like you do other meetings and events in your life. Some days wearing exercise attire can help with making you ready to move when the time permits.

Use Time before Work or Starting Your Day

Set your alarm 30 minutes earlier. Don't be afraid to get up a little earlier and get your workout first thing in the morning. This may be the only time you have available on certain days.

Use Time after Work, at the End of Your Day, or During Your Lunch Hour

Hit the gym in the evening or after you leave the office. Use your lunchtime. Your workout can be a great stress reliever and can be completed in 30 minutes, leaving you time for a light lunch or dinner.

Incorporate Exercise into Your Day

Take the stairs and park in the furthest spot while out and about. Play actively with your kids or grandkids. Housework, gardening, and other activities count. Do your own running around the house rather than having others bring you things.

Incorporate Exercise or Movement into Your Recreation

Find activities that keep you moving on the weekends or in the evenings. Join a team sport or take up a new class. My gym now offers couples dance lessons on Friday nights to give our members something active to do that doesn't feel like a workout. In class we dance, move, play, sweat and have fun.

Recruit a Workout Partner

A workout partner, whether a friend, family member, or personal trainer will help you be accountable for exercising on a regular basis. It is easier to get in your workout if someone is waiting for you or encouraging you to exercise.

Learn to Love Moving

Let working out grow on you. Allow it to become part of your life. Love and enjoy moving because it makes you feel better. Focus on the benefits of becoming stronger, more heart healthy and invigorated. You should be able to enjoy being active; there are so many ways to do it! Find what exercise and movement you enjoy and stick with it.

Fight Fatigue with Fitness

After a draining day, it's probably your mind and not your body that's tired. Try moving to relieve feelings of fatigue and exhaustion. There are physiological and neurological mechanisms that will improve your body and your mind.

Strategy 17

BodyJoy Exercise Product Recommendations

Many people do not have the luxury of belonging to a gym or health club and even those who belong to a gym enjoy having a couple of pieces of equipment at home to use at their convenience. My recommendations are for exercise products that are affordable and can be used by anyone—regardless of ability or age. These are The BodyGym, Stability Balls and a pedometer. With these three affordable products, you will have the ability to perform strength training, cardio, flexibility and balance exercises. And best of all, you can have all the essential workout equipment you need for less than $100!

The BodyGym

The BodyGym is a resistance-training product that eliminates the need for weight plates and several other pieces of heavy workout equipment. It is band training at its finest. It's a simple solution for building and toning muscle, which is a key to losing weight. The BodyGym is a resistance band connected to a lightweight, yet sturdy, plastic bar, with webbing straps attached. You can perform nearly any exercise with the BodyGym that typically requires barbells, dumbbells, and other expensive, heavy, weight training equipment.

The BodyGym bar is an ergonomically designed, lightweight, plastic bar that is simple to assemble and break down for storage or transportation. The BodyGym's webbing straps are an exclusive patent, which contribute to the product's versatility. They can be used as handles or foot straps, depending on the exercise. The straps allow you to train limbs independently. You can perform nearly any exercise with the straps that you would with a dumbbell.

It is a simple, affordable and results-based solution to strength training. If you only buy one product, this should be it. You can also stretch and perform cardio with BodyGym. I have seen countless bodies transform just by using this effective product.

Stability Balls

Stability balls were traditionally utilized for physical therapy. Today, they are an essential component of exercise at any training level. They assist you in improving your core strength, which is the most important strength your body requires.

Your core is where all movement in your body originates. Not only that, but when you perform any activity (walk, run, twist, or bend), your core muscles are hard at work, keeping you aligned and stabilizing your body as your weight shifts. Your body's core is the area around your mid-section and pelvis.

This is where your center of gravity is located. When you have appropriate core stability, the muscles in your pelvis, lower back, hips and abdomen work in harmony. They provide support to your spine for just about any activity. However, if your core is weak, you're susceptible to pain and injury. Individuals with weak core muscles typically experience lower-back pain. Strong core muscles keep your posture correct and protect you from injury.

A strong core provides the stabilization necessary to carry groceries or pick up a child. It protects you while doing high-intensity activities such as running, dancing, and lifting heavy objects. Core strengthening is about working your muscles from the inside out. Stability balls train your core to be strong and supportive to your body's frame and movements.

Whether you're a rehabilitation patient, a beginning exerciser, or the most elite athlete, you can benefit from using a stability ball. Balls can be purchased at most recreational stores or online at *www.mindybuxton.com*. They typically range from $25 to $50. Some even come with an instructional video/CD. I recommend that you have a session with a certified personal trainer before using a stability ball to learn proper form to prevent potential injury from performing movements incorrectly. The trainer can provide you with exercises appropriate for your individual level and ability.

Pedometers

Pedometers measure steps and distances in walking and running. They are battery-operated devices containing a spring-suspended, horizontal lever arm that moves up and down. This motion opens and closes an electrical circuit in response to vertical accelerations of the waist that occur during walking and running. The electronic circuitry accumulates steps and provides a digital display.

Pedometers provide a tangible way to measure recommendations such as taking the stairs instead of the elevator. A pedometer is a good motivator as it allows wearers to strive toward a fixed goal that can be modified, depending on the individual involved. In addition, it does not involve large investments of time or money.

Recent evidence suggests that adults should aim to take 10,000 steps every day. Children and adolescents should aim for approximately 12-14,000 steps a day. However, some people only manage to take about 3,000 steps each day.

The equipment recommended can help you achieve your goals no matter if you're a seasoned exerciser or if you're just getting started. The only catch is that you have to use it! You'll find all three options are exciting and effective methods of improving your body and experiencing body joy. Get your equipment so you can get started today.

Strategy 18

Rest and Recovery

An important part of any fitness program is recovery and resting from the demands placed on your body. Rest is not "doing nothing." It's an active and valuable pastime. You need it to adapt to the mental and physical demands put on your body. Without rest or recovery time, you invite injury, loss of motivation and sickness. Rest revitalizes. Your body receives physical rest through sleep. Your mind receives mental and emotional rest through calm feelings by taking a break from the worry and stress you experience on a regular basis.

So, when life hands us a few empty moments, why do we feel squeamish, uncomfortable and unaccountably lazy? It's our Western perspective that filling every moment is a sign of value and significance. Perhaps we avoid "empty" time so as not to deal with grief, anxiety, guilt, regret and pain. Where do you fit in? Do you equate your worth based on how much you accomplish?

Are you purposefully trying to distract yourself by having an overflowing schedule? Are you doing everything but accomplishing nothing? What good is that? Some emotional eaters fill down time with eating! Many of my clients tend to eat when they feel like they have down time or nothing to do. They feel like they always need to be doing something.

Never resting or clearing out your time is like never emptying out your garbage can, your bladder or your digestive tract. Those are not pretty images. Filling your time with tasks that may not be necessary can hurt you from having your best life.

Is your schedule hindering you from having your best body and life?

In spite of everything you do . . .

- Are you irritable or do you feel frayed?
- Are you bored (oddly enough)?
- Do you feel disconnected from others?
- Are you unable to unwind at night or on vacation?
- Do you have a sense of not being, having or doing enough?

If you can answer "yes" to any of these questions, it is time to flush your schedule and find some empty time to rest, heal, and revitalize.

How do you find rest or empty time?

Prioritize

Which tasks in your schedule will you be glad you did? Which tasks don't matter that much to you? Which will mean nothing? Remember a time when you did something that made you feel good. If something does not offer soulful nourishment or bring you pleasure, it may not be high priority. Of course, we all have responsibilities we must do—like pick your kids up from school, wash your laundry, go to work—just make sure you prioritize around those to include time for yourself.

I sometimes find myself making things harder or more elaborate than they really need to be. My intentions are good, yet I get overwhelmed and pressed for time. Even though I put more details into something to try and make it better, I get more stressed and don't enjoy the moment.

I know I'm a much nicer and happier mom and spouse when I'm accomplishing important tasks and not getting myself worked up over things that won't matter in the end. I often have to remind myself to prioritize. We can't always do everything all at once and that's okay, it's not expected! When you prioritize, focus on what's truly important and let go of the rest.

Protect

When you are able to find empty time, be sure to keep your appointment to relax and rebuild. There will always be something that comes up or something you can find to fill your time. Resist the pressure and understand how much more effective you will be if you are rejuvenated and revitalized. You can accomplish more without getting burned out, you'll feel better, have a more productive mind and experience less stress and sickness. Commit to keep your commitment to find rest or recovery time on a regular basis.

Sometimes you may find yourself unexpectedly in "R & R" time: waiting at the dentist, sitting in traffic, a cancelled appointment, a delayed flight. Here are some ideas that can turn unexpected down time into refreshing experiences.

If you have one minute . . .

Go limp. Settle into the most comfortable position possible. Inhale deeply for 4 to 8 seconds, hold your breath a second or two, and then relax your body and face muscles as you exhale for 4 to 8 seconds. Become aware of what you are feeling. Breathe into your entire diagram. Let your chest rise and fall without using your shoulders to lift your body on the inhale.

Your body will repay the gift of oxygen and relaxation by becoming more calm and energetic. I try to do this in traffic or at my computer or whenever I need a minute to experience calmness. Once I finish straightening my house or in between laundry loads or chasing kids, I plop down and just sit in silence before turning on music or picking up a book. Sometimes one good quiet minute can go a long way in a crazy chaotic day.

If you have five minutes . . .

Jot down a quick "to-do" list, then forget everything and let your mind roam free. Patiently and nonjudgmentally, watch where your mind goes and what it says. Remember a favorite vacation. Recall the details: how things smelled, how the air felt, the warmth of the sun, feelings you experienced.

You can have the benefit of being as refreshed and energized as you did on your vacation without ever going anywhere. I often visit Aruba or Cabo San Lucas in my mind. I recreate the experience of lying on the warm sand with a light ocean breeze brushing my face. For this city girl, there is nothing like a trip to the beach to relax and rejuvenate.

If you have an hour . . .

Find a reason to laugh. Read a book or call your silliest friend. If you are too stressed or sad to laugh, then cry. Both behaviors release physical and emotional tension connecting your mind and body. Laughter has been shown to improve immune function, strengthen relationships, and brighten your mood in almost any situation. You could get a massage (my favorite and most cherished recovery hour), pedicure, facial, listening to music, or take a yoga or pilates class. Find something that will rejuvenate your mind and body.

Strategy 19

Sleep On This . . .

In today's high-stress world, people constantly have stress hormones over-stimulating their bodies. This elevated stress response can lead to many health problems including hypertension, cancer, ulcers, lower-back pain and headaches. Non-exercise variables, including lack of sleep, inadequate nutrition and high stress levels, can significantly affect hormone levels that impact exercise recovery (the rate your body adapts and recovers from your workout), health, and the ability to lose body fat and inches.

Individuals who have chronically high stress levels, inadequate sleep and poor nutrition will not recover and adapt to exercise at the same rate as individuals with optimal levels of stress, sleep and nutrition. This is one explanation of why fat loss and fitness improvement may grind to a halt in some individuals, while other individuals continue adapting and progressing in their exercise programs.

Research indicates that sleep deprivation can lead to an elevation in Cortisol and is harmful to carbohydrate metabolism, increasing the chance of obesity. According to Michael Thorpy, Ph.D., and director of the Sleep Wake Disorders Center at Montefiore Medical Center in New York, "Sleep loss is associated with striking alterations in hormone levels that regulate appetite and may be a contributing factor to obesity. Anyone making a commitment to losing weight should probably consider a parallel commitment to get more sleep." Most individuals benefit from having between eight and ten hours of sleep each night.

Remember the client I mentioned earlier who lost all the inches? An additional factor that influenced her successful change was her sleeping pattern. She began getting more sleep once she quit her job. Both her family practitioner and I attribute part of her success to her body's positive response to getting more sleep.

Things that negatively affect your sleep cycle

- Soda
- Sugar
- Alcohol
- Stress level-find something calming to do at night
- Too much food at night
- Too much protein at night-body has to work hard to digest it, can cause nightmares

Tips for Better Sleep

- Use your bed for sleeping purposes only. Do not use it to work on, read or watch television.
- When you become drowsy, get up and go to bed! Don't allow yourself to doze off on the sofa or in a chair. Listen to your body and get to bed.
- When you can't sleep, try slow breathing techniques and relaxing imagery. If you haven't dozed off within 20 minutes, get up and read or do some type of quiet activity. Go back to bed when you get sleepy.
- Get regular exposure to daylight.
- Sleep experts recommend lying on your back or your side.
- Eliminate any light in your bedroom. Try aiming the alarm clock so it's out of sight.
- Melatonin supplement as a sleep aid. Take between 1-4mg of melatonin as a sleep aid.
- Only take over-the-counter sleep aids on occasion. You can build up a tolerance to them. If you find yourself relying on them, see your doctor.

If you continue to experience interrupted sleep or feel you have insomnia or a related sleeping disorder, see your doctor. I know from experience that sleep affects my results. There are times when I am diligent about getting in my workouts and watching my nutrition, but if I'm not sleeping well or enough I don't see decreases in my body fat or inch loss.

I find that I even eat more as a response to being tired. When I make the necessary changes to get adequate amounts of sleep, I have a much easier time changing my body and seeing improvements. As a mother of two young children who and tend to wake at all hours of the night, I've altered my first client's appointment time to get in more sleep so I can keep my body functioning at its best. I have the ability to set my own hours, so this works for me.

What are some measures you can take to receive the adequate amount of sleep your body needs? Do you need to set a more regular bedtime? Can you take care of some stressful issues so you can sleep more peacefully? Are you drinking caffeine or eating excessive amounts of sugar after 3pm? Is your alarm clock keeping your room lit at night?

List the changes you can make to improve your sleep.

_____

_____

_____

_____

_____

_____

Meals

This is not a plan that will give you a few eating instructions to follow until you get so burned out on restricting calories that you binge and gain more fat than you ever lost. This is not a plan that gives you a month of exercises then leaves you stuck on a plateau. This is the last book you will ever need in order to change your body. It provides you with all you need to know about why dieting will never bring long-term results as well as providing you with a new eating plan for life. Your new eating plan is simple. It is based on two principles: the *quality* of food and the *quantity* of food. So if you're hungry for a realistic, long-term approach to nutrition, dig in!

Strategy 20

Stop Dieting and Start Changing Your Body

My guess is that you've been unable to permanently lose unwanted body fat. Since you haven't found your best body yet, you probably aren't experiencing body joy. You may be among the millions of Americans who diet or take weight-loss supplements. You may have found yourself getting heavier after each new diet attempt. You're not alone. The diet craze has been at the forefront of the weight-loss industry since the 1960s. Several new diet plans emerge each year.

Billions of dollars are spent annually on weight-loss gimmicks and diet programs, yet obesity is the leading cause of preventable death in America. It's one of the most resistant medical conditions to permanent treatment—even harder to cure than cancer.[10] Over 60 percent of the American population has eaten themselves into some degree of obesity and malnutrition by consuming nutritionally inadequate foods.[11] The answer to changing your body is not found in a weight-loss supplement. It takes something other than a diet to create your best body.

The simple truth is: gaining body fat is not something that can just be *cured;* it is something that needs to be *managed.* Your ideal body—once

---

[10]   *McGraw, Dr. Phil, Ultimate Weight Solution, New York: The Free Press, 2003*

[11]   *Chek, Paul, You Are What You Eat—Processed Foods, 2004*

reached—is something you'll need to work at to maintain. This is why diets are unsuccessful. You simply can't eat differently for a few weeks or even months and expect permanent results. Do you know where the concept of the word diet actually comes from? It originates from the Greek word *"dieta." Dieta* means "way of life." It refers to your diet plan or nutrition plan, not the American version of dieting.

Dieting has actually become a "way of life" for countless Americans, but it is a way that robs self-respect, freedom, BodyJoy, peace with food, and happiness. Contrary to what fad diets say, permanent changes do require effort. They require you to make a choice to stop dieting and start living a healthier *dieta.*

Healthy eating can include delicious flavors and simple food choices. It doesn't have to mean less flavor, weird "health foods," or deprivation. Here's some news I think you'll enjoy: If you implement my recommendations, you won't have to give up anything completely. You can eat your dessert or whatever other food *you* love. You will learn how to enjoy it as part of your new, healthier, meal plan. My plan focuses on basic concepts to make it as easy as possible to find your best body and experience body joy.

The Metabolism Factor

Fad diets will never produce long-term effects because of the body's metabolic system. In basic terms, metabolism is the rate at which your body breaks down the nutrients in food to produce energy.

BodyJoy Tip

Did you know that one pound of fat burns only two calories, while one pound of muscle or lean mass burns 50 calories?

Body composition (your lean or muscle mass vs. fat mass) is the primary factor that determines your **resting metabolic rate (RMR)** or the number of calories your body burns at rest, or if you were to merely sit in a chair all day. The higher your fat-free mass (including lean muscle, bones, and organs), the higher your resting metabolic rate will be. Heredity and hormones such as insulin and thyroid are important factors that dictate metabolism. Controllable factors such as stress, caloric intake, exercise and medications also play a role. By improving your eating habits and your exercise and movement, you can improve your metabolism!

What Dieting Does

Most diets require excessive calorie restrictions, which ultimately leave us larger than we were before we dieted. When you restrict calories excessively, you will experience a five to ten percent drop in your resting metabolic rate. It slows down to store what you eat. This is your body's way to conserve energy when food is in short supply. It's a survival mechanism we're wired with.

Food affects your resting metabolic rate in terms of total calories or *how much* you eat (not *what* you eat). The longer you starve your body—by eating too few calories—the more calories your body will store. As you begin to eat a more realistic amount of calories, you will notice weight gain since your body is in storing or survival mode. This is the reason most people end up weighing more after they end a diet than they did before they started it. Your body will put itself in survival mode whenever you drastically restrict your calories.

There is no way to metabolically trick your body. Ultimately, there is no way to avoid gaining weight after you diet. This is why I can say diets don't work long term. **Ninety-five percent** of the people who lose weight regain it (and sometimes even additional weight). Diets are dangerous, lower self-respect, cause fatigue, deplete energy, increase preoccupation with food and disrupt normal eating.

Most diets are not even based on science or common sense, although they may give that impression in their advertising. Most diet regimens provide short-term success and long-term health consequences. The American Dietetic Association states, "When people lose weight on the Atkins' Diet (and nearly all other diets), it's only because they are consuming fewer calories."

Fad diets severely restrict calories and place the focus on a single food element (such as high protein or low carbs) leaving out important weight loss management strategies like portion control, serving sizes, variety and moderation. When you move away from diets and focus on eating for health, you establish a sound nutritional plan that will allow for inch and fat loss over the short-term and long-term maintenance once your goal is achieved.

Inch and fat percentage loss can be achieved without adversely affecting your metabolic rate, by moderately reducing your calorie intake and increasing your activity level simultaneously. For example, it takes cutting out 3,500 calories to lose a pound. If your goal is to lose one pound per week, you need to cut 500 calories a day. You can cut 250 calories each day by reducing your portion sizes at meals, and can burn an additional 250 calories each day by moderately increasing your amount of exercise.

BodyJoy Tip

The only successful way to lose body fat and inches, be healthy and avoid regaining weight is through moderate (not excessive) caloric changes.

An analysis published in the journal Science illustrated that a deficit of 200-260 calories per day is all that would be needed to prevent gaining fat in 90 percent of the population.[12] A decrease of this many calories is equivalent to a modest drop in food intake (such as cutting out one candy bar or Krispy Cream glazed donut) and walking an extra 3-6 miles over a 1- to 2-hour period every day. You don't have to starve yourself to experience results!

Moderate changes result in long-term fat loss and improved health. If you lose one pound a week for the next two months, you will be eight to nine pounds thinner—which is at least one pant size. In contrast, you could diet by excessively restricting your calories and lose eight to ten pounds (of muscle and water) in only two weeks. Doing this typically results in being 10 to 12 pounds heavier within a month from when you stop dieting. By restricting your caloric intake, you may lose weight faster, but the chances you will keep the weight off long-term are slim. If you lose more than two pounds per week, plan on that weight (plus some additional pounds) coming back.

Here's an excellent example how moderate changes result in long-term results. I have a training client who made one simple focus change which eliminated the way she use to struggle with her most tempting food. This client was a classic dieter who ended up binge eating with her favorite food—chips. When she dieted she would not allow herself to eat chips. She never bought them and she restricted herself from eating them when she went out to restaurants. She viewed chips as a "bad" food. The severe restrictions she placed on chips always ended up back firing. When she would break down and eat them, she ate chips uncontrollably.

---

[12]   *Science, August 1, 2003*

This client has worked through a number of "diet mentality" issues, changing her perception from thinking foods are "bad" to food is "neutral" and not placing severe restrictions on what she can or can't eat. Once she decided to change her unrealistic restrictions off chips and allowed herself to have them when she felt like eating them, the deprivating urgency to binge and devourer all the chips she could suddenly disappeared.

Once the negative association was changed into a positive one, knowing she was allowed to eat chips, they became non-threatening to her inch and fat loss goals. She now can keep a bag of chips in her house without needing to eat the entire bag in one sitting. In fact, she can go months at a time before finishing her bag at home. This is a completely different scenario compared to how she used to experience chips as a dieter. By merely changing her focus from deprivation to entitlement, she found peace and control over a dieting element, which she struggled with for years.

It's sometimes difficult or scary to change your mentality about food. The benefits are well worth it. Many individuals are surprised at how a little thing like "forbidding chips" can affect their goals in wanting to improve their bodies. Before you can change your body, you must make some changes to your nutrition. Change doesn't mean deprivation, restrictions or punishments. It can mean simply altering amounts and still enjoying the foods you love.

You need to understand that high calories and huge portions give you the body you have now. Restrictions and bingeing from dieting could be keeping you stuck. Keep in mind; you are entitled to any food you want. Let go of sabotaging restrictions and watch your food obsessions and cravings lessen. Small changes or adaptations to how you eat can be accommodating to your healthier lifestyle. These changes can be without struggle or conflict. You can find a place for any food with this healthy eating plan.

Resistance Training

Resistance training or strength training is the most effective way to build and preserve lean muscle mass. Each pound of muscle you gain can raise your resting metabolic rate to burn more calories per day.[13] The more

---

[13]   *Gary Foster, Ph. D, University of Pennsylvania*

lean muscle mass you have, the more overall calories you will burn at rest as well as during exercise. Fat and inch loss can be accelerated when you focus on building muscle.

Before I became a trainer I thought that in order to lose fat I needed to do more cardio exercise. I was surprised at how much easier it was for me to lose body fat and keep it off once I began strength training. Not only did my fat percentage decrease, but I didn't have to spend as much time doing cardio exercise because I had more muscle mass burning calories for me.

Varied Cardio Intensity

Short-term metabolic boosts can come from high-intensity cardiovascular activity. This is known as interval training. Your metabolic rate increases 20-30 percent depending on intensity while exercising. The higher the intensity, the more calories you will burn during exercise. It's important to vary your cardiovascular activity if you expect to lose body fat.

Don't get too caught up in keeping your heart rate around 60-65 percent all the time (this is typically known as the fat-burning zone). If you keep your intensity varied and hit high intensity, moderate intensity and lower intensity periods you will see your metabolic rate improve. There are metabolic benefits to doing cardio activity in all three zones.

Medications

Medications such as those used to treat depression and bi-polar disorder have been shown to lower metabolism. Talk to your doctor about the side effects that your medications may be causing you. If you feel your medications are affecting you, see if there are alternatives without negative side effects.

Myths Regarding Metabolism

You can have more of an effect on your metabolism than you may think. Most factors that increase your metabolism are factors you have control over. Don't use these four myths as excuses:

1. *Heavy people have slow metabolisms*

Size does not determine your metabolic rate: it's your body composition (fat mass vs. lean mass). You can take two people who have identical looking physiques and they can have drastically different metabolisms. If you have a naturally slow metabolism, gaining weight is not inevitable, although it may be tougher—but not impossible—to lose. Whatever your metabolic rate, you can raise it to some extent through eating appropriately, exercising and building lean muscle mass in order to lose body fat percentage and inches.

2. *Age affects your Resting Metabolic Rate (RMR)*

Age only affects your RMR 2-3 percent per *decade.* I have clients who've been able to look and feel better in their 40s and 50s than they did in their 20s. It wasn't until I reached my third decade (and had had two children) that I was able to find my best body. Age is not as much to blame as we may think, it's muscle loss from a lack of activity as we age that contributes to a lower metabolic rate. It's never too late to start exercising and eating better. Whatever your age, you can prevent that small metabolic decrease each decade by exercising on a regular basis and by being aware of your nutrition.

3. *Spicy foods raise your RMR*

Research shows that eating spicy food does not affect metabolic rates enough to see a decrease at your waistline. With regard to your metabolism, there is no reason to increase your intake of spicy foods or seasonings.

BodyJoy Tip

Take it slow and steady. You'll be able to lose fat, maintain muscle mass and develop realistic eating habits you can easily stick with for life.

4. *Fat-burner supplements*

Supplements that promote elevating your metabolism or burning fat do not work long-term. They're expensive and potentially dangerous. There is a lack of evidence on how they affect your body long-term.

There are a number of deaths and health issues that can be linked to taking these types of supplements. The sad thing is, you won't know how they will affect you until you have a negative side effect. These are not worth the risk. You are much better off going for a brisk walk or getting to the gym to cause an elevation in your metabolic rate.

There are methods available to determine your personal resting metabolic rate. If you are interested in being tested or having your RMR determined visit the website *www.mindybuxton.com*. Knowing your exact RMR can greatly assist you in knowing how many calories you can eat and how many calories you'll need to burn while reaching your goals. These assessments generally take from five to ten minutes and require you to fast and avoid exercise within four hours of testing.

Strategy 21

The BodyJoy Nutrition Plan: Whole Foods First, Processed Foods Less and Appropriate Portions

Eating is something you have to do every day. It is essential for survival. It's important to eat to live, not live to eat. Food is a source of energy that sustains our daily activities. I like to keep things simple and focus on two main elements of food: the *quality* and the *quantity*.

Your body is the vehicle that you use to accomplish your activities. Would you ever fill the gas tank of your car with sand or water? Of course not! This is what you are doing to your body when you fuel it with highly processed foods. This new plan will help you understand why it's important to use only the finest quality of foods as fuel to keep your body fit and healthy. You will also learn correct quantities in order to see physical changes and have adequate energy to perform activities.

Food fads have led us to believe that carbohydrates are bad and proteins are good. In years past, fat was bad and carbohydrates were good. Both scenarios led people to think they could eat as much of the "good" food as they wanted with no consequences. These methods have failed to provide permanent fat loss. You need to learn to eat enough food to sustain energy and bring about physical changes when desired. This isn't done by starving yourself, severely restricting calories, or by avoiding entire food groups.

The typical American eats:

- Small amounts of whole foods
- Large amounts of processed sugars and grains
- Excessively high-fat fast foods
- Extremely large portion sizes
- Excessive amounts of animal protein and fat

This type of eating is loaded with high calories and lacks nutritional value. It's a lifestyle that increases your risk of obesity, heart disease, hypertension, high cholesterol, type II diabetes, and other diseases. The majority of calories come from high-fat and high-sugar products that are harmful to your best body and health. Not only are these food choices unhealthy, they are typically eaten in ridiculously high amounts. (Sand into the gas tank!)

What does your current nutrition plan look like?

- _____ amounts of vegetables and fruits
- _____ amounts of whole grains
- _____ amounts of water
- _____ amounts of *healthy* proteins
- _____ amounts of healthy oils and fats
- _____ amounts of refined and processed foods
- _____ amounts of hydrogenated fats and trans-fats
- _____ amounts of preservatives and additives

The BodyJoy Nutrition Plan is simple: eat whole foods first, processed foods less frequently and appropriate portion sizes. Rather than categorizing food by macronutrients (carbohydrates, proteins, and fats) this plan focuses on food by assessing its nutritional and caloric values. You will learn to eat the most nutrients for the fewest calories. You will learn to shift your focus from processed food choices and to concentrate on increasing whole food choices. *This allows you to feel full on fewer calories while you lose inches and body fat long-term.*

There are only two rules to follow:

1. Eat nutritious whole foods first and processed foods less frequently.
2. Use appropriate servings or portion sizes when you eat.

BodyJoy Tip

"Research has shown no better way to slow or even reverse the progress of aging itself and of all the age-related degenerative conditions than through the combination of aerobic, and strength-building exercise and a balanced, nutritious diet."

—Nutrition expert Dr. Irwin Rosenberg

If you follow the concepts outlined, you will have no need to diet. You will not have to go without your favorite foods; you'll just learn to enjoy them in different amounts. These guidelines are specific, yet flexible enough for you to include those foods you personally enjoy. You will learn the importance of essential nutrients, variety and the principle of moderation.

It's imperative that you optimize your dietary choices in order to achieve your best body and a high quality life. Our Western lifestyle demands convenience. Processed foods typically provide this because they are already bagged and ready to go. They are also typically sweet and easy to eat in a mindless manner. There are healthy, more nutritious alternatives to fast food. You just need to incorporate healthier substitutes for the not-so-healthy foods you currently use. Healthy nutrition can provide a feeling of fullness that lasts longer than the usual sugar rush you get from a candy bar. Smart food choices can also make the difference between hitting 3pm sluggishness or having lasting energy throughout the day.

You'll be able to modify your food habits if your focus is on what you should be eating, not on what you can't have. This food plan does not require you to never eat processed food again. It allows it in moderation and in correct amounts. If you can learn to master this, you can be in control of your figure and experience body joy for the rest of your life.

Why Whole Foods?

As we say "Goodbye" to diets, we say "Hello" to whole foods. What are whole foods? Whole foods are foods that are closest to their original or natural state. They are simple foods or foods in their most simple form. They contain significant quantities of vitamins, minerals, fiber and phytochemicals. Vitamins and minerals are essential nutrients necessary for growth and development. Phytochemicals have disease fighting properties. Fiber is necessary for proper digestive functioning, has the potential for fighting certain diseases and is critical in helping you feel full. These important nutrients, in their original state, are found in whole foods.

Fiber

Fiber is the part of plant food the body can't digest completely. Your inability to digest fiber provides health benefits. Waste products pass through the body quicker when you have a diet rich in fiber, providing less time for harmful substances to bind to the lining of your intestines. Fiber helps control blood-sugar levels and can make you feel full before you've eaten too many calories. Processed and refined foods are generally stripped or reduced of their fiber content, allowing you to eat more calories before you begin to feel full. The more fiber in your meals, the more full you will feel.

Phytochemicals

Phytochemicals are plant-based nutrients. There are thousands of phytochemicals found in plant foods. They provide significant health benefits. Phytochemicals are the substances that give fruits and vegetables their vibrant colors. They also are the compounds that give some foods their pungent or burning taste. Phytochemicals have been shown to protect against cancer, heart disease, and other illnesses. They may improve lung function, slow the aging process, and reduce problems associated with diabetes. A diet rich in a variety of fruits, vegetables, and whole grains is the most reliable way to receive phytonutrients.

Vitamins and Minerals

Vitamins are essential compounds that enable chemical reactions in the body to occur. While vitamins themselves do not provide energy, they help release the energy found in food. Minerals are essential chemicals that are necessary for chemical reactions and they form the body's structure. They are necessary for proper growth and development and they regulate many of the body's processes.

Whole foods are packed with nutrients important for optimal health and well-being. By eating more whole foods, you have the ability to eat more food, consume fewer calories, and be healthier. **Consuming whole foods that are lower in calories than their processed counterparts allows you to eat more food without gaining inches or body fat.**

Even though whole foods are more nutrient dense, they still need to be eaten in response to your body's needs. Eating more calories in whole foods than your body needs will lead to gaining body fat and inches.

The advantages to whole foods include:

1. You can generally eat a greater quantity of many whole foods.
2. You can feel fuller and more satisfied on fewer calories.
3. You receive more nutrients.
4. Your cravings tend to decrease.
5. You're energy level can become more constant.

The BodyJoy Nutrition plan consists of:

- Large amounts of vegetables and fruits
- Large amounts of whole grains
- Adequate amounts of water
- Moderate amounts of healthy proteins
- Moderate amounts of healthy oils and fats
- Low amounts of refined and processed foods
- Low amounts of hydrogenated fats and trans-fats
- Low amounts of preservatives and additives

The BodyJoy nutrition plan is a "flexitarian" approach. It's more well-rounded than a strictly vegetarian diet, yet it's healthier than the typical carnivorous diet. This nutrition plan is mainly whole-foods based, but includes healthy protein and dairy in moderation. The Western way of eating tends to center meals around meat rather than placing the emphasis on vegetables, fruits and whole foods.

My plan places meat in the category of healthy sources of protein, but recommends you eat it less frequently than the typical American. This plan does not exclude anything as forbidden or prohibited, it just alters the amounts of certain foods.

You can begin adapting aspects of the plan now in a way that works for you. It may be three days a week, every other day, or only one meal a day. Perhaps you will be able to switch over to this meal plan completely.

The guidelines are for healthy fat and inch loss and to help you feel and function at your best. Any modifications to your nutrition habits are better than none! Every adaptation, no matter how small or insignificant you may think it is, will help you see results.

Nutrient Categories

The following section outlines essential nutrients necessary for optimal heath and for achieving your best body. Each category provides a food continuum of the healthiest choices first, followed by the least healthy choices for that category.

Water

Water is essential! Your body is made up of approximately 70 percent water. Water plays an important role in all aspects of metabolism, carrying nutrients to their intended destination and wastes out of the body. Water is also necessary for joint lubrication and for temperature regulation.

BodyJoy Tip

Why is water consumption so important? It suppresses the appetite, assists the body in metabolizing stored fat, reduces fat deposits or the appearance of cellulite, relieves fluid retention problems, hydrates the skin, reduces sodium build up, helps maintain proper muscle tone, rids the body of waste and toxins, and relieves constipation.

Each function of your body is linked to the efficient flow of water. Water is lost on a daily basis through respiration, elimination, and perspiration. When your body is dehydrated, cells can't function properly and you have decreased energy.

Fruits and vegetables are an important source of water. The rest of your body's fluid needs should come from drinking water. You are already in a dehydrated state once you begin to feel thirsty. Since thirst is not an adequate indicator of when you need water, your goal should be to drink enough water to avoid ever feeling thirsty.

I recommend drinking at least one-half a gallon of water each day (8-10 eight-ounce glasses). If your activity level increases, you may need to increase the amount of water you ingest. If this amount sounds overwhelming, start by adding one or two glasses a day. It is much better to gradually increase your intake rather than not change your hydration habits at all. In my experience, *drinking an adequate amount of water is one of the most overlooked aspects of fat loss.*

Since water is a natural resource, perhaps we take its effects for granted. Get into the habit of always having a water bottle with you whether you are on-the-go, at home, or at the office. Drink your water as often as you can. **Sometimes we respond to thirst with food rather than with a beverage.** Before you start eating, make sure you have been drinking enough water and quench your thirst by drinking water.

With regard to other beverages

By reducing the amount of soda and alcohol you drink, and increasing your water intake, it is easy to reduce the number of calories in your diet. Soda and alcohol should be used in strict moderation or avoided completely—even diet sodas. Water is the best beverage for maintaining hydration and should be your drink of choice when it comes to fat loss and health.

BodyJoy Tip

As little as a 10 percent loss of water can cause symptoms such as difficulty concentrating, dizziness, muscle spasms, and failing kidney function.

I have had clients who try to wean themselves from drinking sodas by replacing soda with juice. They get frustrated when they do not see their body fat drop. Juice contains a high amount of calories from sugar. Drink juices in moderation. A serving size of juice is only 6 ounces. If you need some flavor in your water, try adding lemon or lime juice to it.

Vegetables

BodyJoy Tip

High-heat methods of cooking such as steaming, stir-frying, and microwaving vegetables preserve more nutrients.

Vegetables are low in calories and high in fiber, vitamins, minerals, and phytochemicals to help reduce your risk of heart disease and certain types of cancers. Their fiber content helps you feel full and aids in weight loss.

Vegetables should be the focus of your meal plan. The greater the variety of vegetables you include, the higher the nutrients you will receive.

By focusing on getting in all the vegetables you're advised to eat each day, you automatically weed out opportunities to eat high-calorie, low-nutrient dense foods. Vegetables should be eaten in abundance on a daily basis. There is a world of vegetable out there you probably haven't even tried yet. Be flexible and experimental.

Vegetable Continuum

(From healthiest to least healthy.)

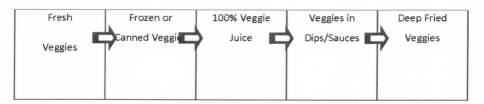

Fresh Veggies	Frozen or Canned Veggies	100% Veggie Juice	Veggies in Dips/Sauces	Deep Fried Veggies

Ways to incorporate vegetables:

- Eating them plain or raw of course!
- Dipping them in hummus or salsa
- Steaming and sprinkling them with herbs for flavor
- Roasting them for a few minutes with olive oil and seasonings or herbs drizzled on top
- Adding them to egg white omelets
- Pureeing them and adding into recipes
- Blending them and adding into shakes or smoothies (I love spinach in my protein shakes!)
- Preparing a large mixed salad or soup and keeping it on hand to use through the week
- Using some of your pre-made salad to make a quick vegetable stir-fry

Fruits

Fruits are typically higher in calories than vegetables and are also rich in nutrients. Different fruits offer different nutrients and all are important to consume. Fruits should be used often in your diet, not just as snacks and desserts. Try adding them to salads and entrées or enjoy them as a dish. Like vegetable, fruits require little preparation time if eaten in their simplest form, and are almost always available. Fresh whole fruits can be a source of fiber that fills you up, not out.

BodyJoy Tip

The key to both vegetables and fruits is to eat a variety of them to receive the most nutrients available. After all, variety is the spice of life! Always keep a bowl of fresh fruit or vegetables on your counter. The more accessible they are, the more you will eat them. Both food groups are convenient and easy to take on-the-go.

Fruit Continuum

Fresh Whole Fruit	Frozen Fruit	Dried Fruit	Canned Fruit	100% Fruit Juice	Apple Pie
	No sugar added	No sugar added	Light syrup or no sugar added		

Whole Grains

Whole Grains are rich in fiber and help reduce the risk of heart disease and diabetes. Grains are essentially seeds that are made up of three main components: the bran, the endosperm and the germ. The bran, or outer shell, protects the seed and provides fiber, B vitamins and some trace minerals. Most of the inner body of the seed is the endosperm, which is rich in protein and carbohydrates.

The germ composes the remaining part of the seed and contains vitamin E as well as other antioxidants and B vitamins. Processed grains, such as white flour, have both the bran and germ removed from the grain. Although some vitamins and minerals have been added back into enriched flours, rices or grains, they still don't have as many nutrients as the "whole" option, and they don't provide nearly as much fiber.

It is important to recognize that many food items say wheat or grain on their labels, but unless the label says "100%," "whole," and unless it is the first item listed in the ingredients, it is a processed imitation. Since whole grains, flours and brown rices aren't stripped of their fiber and are more filling, and more flavorful, smaller portions of them can help you feel satisfied.

Grain Continuum

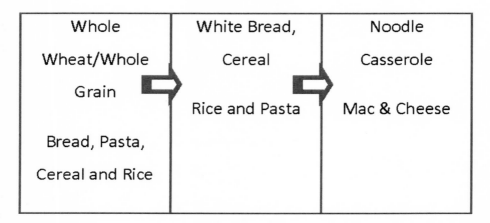

Healthy Proteins (nuts, seeds, legumes, fish, eggs, soy products, poultry and meat)

There is no question high-quality protein is essential for growth and repair of your body. There are several ways to obtain adequate amounts of protein without eating large amounts of meat or poultry. This can be achieved by eating nuts, seeds, legumes (all whole foods by the way!), fish, eggs, and soy products. When meats are the central focus of your diet, you run the risk of eating high saturated fat and cholesterol and thereby increasing your risk of elevated blood lipids that lead to cardiovascular disease. Higher fat intake also leads to higher calories.

BodyJoy Tip

Substitute quick or old-fashioned oats for up to one third of the flour called for in recipes for baked goods.

BodyJoy Tip

The American Institute for Cancer Research says 40 studies have linked regular consumption of whole grains with a 10 to 60 percent lower risk of certain cancers.

With this nutrient group, focus on eating a few *different sources every day*. Rather than having meat and poultry a few times each day, try eating fish, legumes, seeds, nuts, soy, or eggs in place of one or two of your typical meat servings.

Example:

- *Egg whites* for breakfast
- *Nuts* as part of a snack
- *Beans and/or tofu* in salad (replacing chicken for lunch)
- *Edema me* as a snack or side dish
- *Fish* entrée for dinner.

BodyJoy Tip
When selecting meats, choose those labeled "lean" or "very lean." "Select" and "choice" grades are leaner than "prime."

Seeds and nuts are high in protein, fiber and essential fats. Almonds and sesame seeds are great sources of calcium. They are convenient snacks and easy additions to soups, salads and a variety of meals. These foods are higher in calories and healthy fats, so they should be eaten moderately while working on fat-loss goals. The healthiest types of seeds and nuts are whole and/or raw. Keep in mind a serving is 6-12 almonds. Count out your servings of any seeds or nuts. They're so easy to overeat!

Seeds Continuum

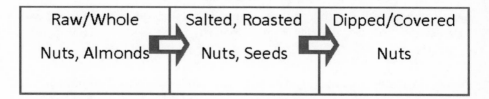

Raw/Whole Nuts, Almonds	Salted, Roasted Nuts, Seeds	Dipped/Covered Nuts

Meats and fish contain quality protein and iron. In addition to protein, meats contain substantial amounts of the B vitamins. Many fish choices are high in essential omega fatty acids. *Eggs* are high in protein but contain little iron. Some eggs are even fortified with Omega3.

Legumes (peas and beans) are high in fiber and a good source of protein. Just one cup of beans gives you half the amount of fiber you need in a day. Their hormone-like compounds may help reduce cholesterol and fight some cancers. They are higher in calories than fruits and vegetables, but, like seeds and nuts, they are filling and easy to add to soups, salads and other meals. Black-eyed peas, black beans, pinto and navy beans are all good sources of calcium.

Soy products are also included in this category. They are often used to make a variety of meat substitutes. They contain no cholesterol, little saturated fat, low sodium and large amounts of fiber. (Most, such as veggie burgers, sausages and ground meat substitutes, taste just as good as the real thing. Try them out on your family—they probably won't even notice a difference.)

Healthy Oils and Fats

While fats have been deemed "bad" food, fats play an important role in nutrition. Fats provide a concentrated source of energy for the body, insulate body tissues, and transport fat-soluble vitamins. It is well known that eating many foods that are high in fat, particularly ones with too much saturated fat and dietary cholesterol, can contribute to the development of clogged and narrowed arteries and excess body fat.

I advise you to eat less saturated fat, tropical oils like coconut and palm, and trans fats. *This means cutting down on high-fat foods, processed foods, and baked goods containing hydrogenated oils.*

Monounsaturated fats are healthier fats. They are liquid at room temperature and become more solid when refrigerated. Monounsaturated fats can be found in olive, canola, almond and peanut oils and may lower LDL (bad) cholesterol levels without lowering the protective HDL (good) cholesterol.

Polyunsaturated fats are liquid at room temperature and remain liquid when refrigerated. Polyunsaturated fats are found in corn, soybean, safflower, flaxseed, and sunflower oils. Polyunsaturated fats may lower LDL cholesterol, but, if used in large quantities, may also lower HDL cholesterol levels. Omega 3 fatty acids and Omega 6 fatty acids are specific polyunsaturated fats that are considered essential and must be obtained from food. You should focus on getting your healthy oils and fats from monounsaturated and polyunsaturated fats.

BodyJoy Tip

What is edema me? Edema me is a soy bean that looks similar to a sugar snap pea. It's the least processed and closest edible product from the natural soy plant itself. You can enjoy edema me steamed and served in their own pods, shelling them as you eat. Edema me is high in protein and is a quick-to prepare side dish or appetizer suitable for today's modern lifestyle. You can find them in the freezer section of your grocery store. (My children and my husband loves them!)

Dairy

Milk and its byproducts are also sources of calcium and protein. Adequate calcium is necessary for proper bone formation and the prevention of osteoporosis. Although dairy products are high in calcium, calcium is also found in certain green vegetables and a variety of beans. Many Americans eat excessive amounts of dairy products: putting cheese on every sandwich and burger, covering other foods with cream and cheese-based sauces and melting grated cheese over everything they can.

Did you know the Food Guide Pyramid recommends only two to three servings per day? That equates to one glass of milk, ½ cup of plain yogurt, and a dice-sized cheese square. Many of us need to eat less of this category or make healthier choices from this food group.

Whole milk products are high in fat—including saturated fat. They should be used sparingly to decrease the risk of elevated blood lipids. Low-fat and skim milk products are the best choices when selecting dairy products. Cheeses are high in sodium and saturated fat. They should be used sparingly and in appropriate amounts.

Dairy Continuum

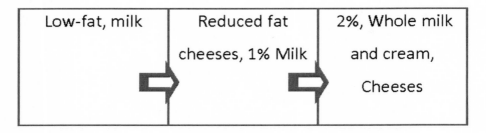

| Low-fat, milk | Reduced fat cheeses, 1% Milk | 2%, Whole milk and cream, Cheeses |

Processed Foods

BodyJoy Tip

If you're trying to lose body fat, lose the soda (even if it's diet)!

Processed foods are foods that have gone through multiple steps for food preservation and flavor enhancement. These are foods that have added sugars, fats and chemicals. The treatments to processed foods enable them to have a longer shelf life and withstand shipping and handling.

All processed foods are not "bad" foods. It's just that they have become so prevalent in our daily diet, replacing foods that contribute essential vitamins and minerals. If you consume a majority of your nutrition from processed foods, you are replacing essential nutrients with empty calories. Those empty calories increase your fat percentage and leave you malnourished. It's a bizarre concept to think we can be overweight and malnourished at the same time.

BodyJoy Tip

In 1997, The World Cancer Research Fund issued a report that found **sixty to seventy percent** *of all cancers can be prevented by staying physically active, not smoking, and most importantly, by following the report's number one dietary recommendation: "Choose predominately plant-based diets rich in a variety of vegetables, fruits, and legumes, and minimally processed starchy staple foods."*

If you are trying to lose inches and body fat, processed foods should be eaten sparingly—not every day at every meal. These foods are high in calories and low in nutrient values. Eating fewer processed foods provides several important health benefits: reduced blood pressure, lower incidence of coronary heart disease, obesity, type II diabetes, kidney and gallstones, and even some forms of cancers. Did you know the U.S. Surgeon General's Report on Nutrition and Health says that two-thirds of United States mortality is diet-related?[14]

BodyJoy Tip

Food scientists have determined how to manipulate the part of your brain that controls food cravings. By adding or subtracting certain nutrients from foods, they can manipulate your sense of hunger and satiety. It's believed that adding excess fat, sugar and salt to a food tends to make people overeat.

Most processed foods have high amounts of sodium. Sodium has an even greater effect on your calcium stores than excess protein does. Many processed foods block your body's ability to maintain calcium. Fortified breads and pastas have been stripped of their fiber and nutrients and only a small amount of their nutrients get added back in. If you find yourself craving a piece of white bread or roll, go ahead and eat it. Just make sure you are enjoying their whole-grain counterparts most of the time. The same rule applies to processed sugars. Eat them sparingly since they have little nutritional value and are high in calories. Stay true to serving sizes and you can enjoy them without gaining unwanted fat.

If you are one who adds sugar to most of your foods, try to find healthier replacements to flavor your meals. Fresh and dried fruits are healthy toppers for cereals, oatmeal, and some desserts. Raisins, bananas, and berries are good choices. Rather than thinking of doing without the sugar,

---

[14]   Robbins, John The Food Revolution, pg. 93

think, "What can I use instead of sugar or sugar substitutes?" Fresh slices of fruit, dried fruit, raisins, nuts or seeds can all add flavor and replace high calorie added sugar. I drizzle Agave Nectar over oatmeal, toast and even over steamed vegetables such as green beans. It tastes like honey, it's natural and it's low glycemic.

BodyJoy Tip

Rather than using salt, butter, cream sauces or other high-calorie, unhealthy seasonings, spreads or dressings, try adding fresh salsa or herbs for flavor or as toppings.

Strategy 22

Surprise . . . It's all About the Size!

Now that you know about food quality, let's talk food quantity! Fat loss and successful body maintenance is not a matter of carbohydrates, proteins, or fats; it is a matter of TOTAL calories or food *quantity*. In all the diet frenzy, people have forgotten the basic principle that *calories in must equal calories out in order to maintain their size*. It's as simple as that! In order **to lose fat and inches you must eat fewer** *calories than you burn* with daily activities and exercise. In fact, one of the simplest nutrition changes you can start with is changing your current portion sizes to these recommended portion sizes.

Correct portion size is essential to fat loss. It affects how many calories you're getting. In my personal training experience, it's the most important factor to changing your figure. *This is the most important weight-loss and inch loss element of the BodyJoy plan.* With this plan, I hope to educate you enough that you can eat any type of food you want and still lose fat because you will be conscious of your portion sizes.

The recommended number of servings in this plan may sound like a lot of food, but portion sizes may be smaller than you realize. It's important to pay attention to your food quantity, serving, or portion size. Sometimes it is the difference between a healthy meal and a fattening one! Your life does not need to be consumed with food, or counting calories, but you do need to be aware of how much you eat so you can achieve your best body and enjoy the benefits of improved health.

When food is eaten in moderate amounts, there is room for your favorite dessert, chocolate every day, or one of your mother's hot, homemade rolls. Foods low in nutrients and high in calories may still be part of your nutrition, they just need to play a smaller roll to the healthier, nutrient dense choices. If you love chocolate, have a piece on occasion. Just make sure you stick to a serving size, and then opt for something healthier if you're still hungry. Eat it without feeling guilty because it's not forbidden. By having one serving, you can afford to enjoy it without gaining body fat.

Chocolate happens to be my "thing". I will never go without chocolate. That's just how it is for me. However, the way I eat it now is different than how I used to enjoy it. I upgraded from quantity to quality and down sized my calories! I buy expensive, European, chocolate truffles. I always have them in my house. I keep them in my cabinet with my bills and old receipts (not my pantry where I can see them all day). When I need a chocolate fix, I go to the cabinet and get a truffle. They are individually wrapped, so I don't need to get the entire package down. Despite the fact, I am too cheap to eat $3 of chocolate in one sitting versus a $.50 candy bar (approximately 250 calories), the truffles are so rich, satisfying and delicious, and I only need one (70 calories) or two to feel gratification.

When I buy the higher quality chocolate, I don't need as much of it to feel satisfied. Now, eating a candy bar just isn't appealing to me as one square or truffle of the finer quality chocolate that I *love*. I eat less of it and feel more satisfied! With my chocolate, I consciously practice mindful eating. Indulging in the "real deal" when it comes to chocolate also translates into consuming less additives, colorings and imitation ingredients that you find in most candy bars and chocolate products. You are still entitled to eat your favorite food, you may just need to find a smarter, healthier way to enjoy it! This is what works for me. What will work for you?

I have seen a number of my training clients change their bodies by simply adjusting the *amount* of food or portion sizes they eat. I have a client named Terry who trained with me for several months without seeing inch or body fat losses. He worked out with me once a week and on his own at least three times. We concluded his exercise was at a decent intensity and duration, but his nutrition was keeping him from seeing results.

My client's life demanded him to eat out at least two meals each day, sometimes three. Since preparing his own meals was not an option, we decided he needed to focus on the amount of food he was eating. He began monitoring his serving sizes and following my suggested portion sizes guidelines. He ate only the designated amount each meal and took the rest home for leftovers or let the restaurant throw it out. He also shared entrees and closely monitored the amount of dressings or sauces he put on his food. The next month we assessed his measurements and body fat, his numbers finally began to change for the better. In one month of monitoring his portions, he lost one and a half percent body fat, six pounds, and four inches over all.

BodyJoy Tip

Read labels to be aware of a single serving size. Be realistic about servings!
If the label says a serving is three pieces and you eat 20—do the math!

When you pay attention to the amounts of food you eat, you don't have to worry about excessive body fat. Americans typically get too many calories by simply eating too much food. Unfortunately, because more of us are eating in restaurants, we are accustomed to eating larger portions than we really need or should have. It's important to remember a serving size isn't the amount you put on your plate, it's the amount of food defined by specific measurements.

This plan makes it easy and convenient to estimate portions. You don't have to bother with weighing your food if you can estimate by the size guidelines provided. Here are the guidelines to follow.

You only need to remember two sizes. It's best to consider an average portion size:

For foods

- The size of your palm
- ½ cup

For dressings or spreads

- The size of your thumb
- 1 Tablespoon

Vegetables

This may include a handful of raw vegetables, 1/2 cup of cooked vegetables, or 1/2 cup of vegetable juice.

Fruit

This may include a medium apple, ½ large apple, ½ cup of no sugar added or 100% fruit juice, a small banana or ½ cup cut fruit bits or pieces.

Whole Grains

This may include ½ cup of hot cereal or dry cereal, ½ cup rice, 1 small slice of whole wheat/grain bread or ½ slice of a large piece.

Healthy Proteins

This may include 12 almonds, handful of raw seeds, or handful of mixed raw nuts. Small chicken breast, one egg or two egg whites. ½ cup beans or lentils, small cut of steak or pork, ½ cut or medium or large piece, 1 tablespoon hummus or 1 tablespoon peanut butter, ½ cup of cooked beans, ½ cup of tofu or temph, or ½ cup of soymilk.

BodyJoy Tip

It's easy to eat huge amounts of seeds and nuts if you are watching TV or have an open container of them at your desk or computer. Be smart and separate them into serving-size baggies so that once that serving is gone, you are done eating them.

Dairy

½ cup low fat milk, ½ cup low fat yogurt or cottage cheese, 1 tablespoon cheese cube, 1 *thin* slice of cheese (size of palm for sandwiches), 1 individual package of string cheese.

Healthy Oils

1 tablespoon olive oil, 1 tablespoon butter, 1 tablespoon flax seed or oil, 1 tablespoon canola oil.

Processed Foods

BodyJoy Tip

When in doubt of a serving size, minimize rather than super size. Did you know that the average takeout muffin is typically five times the size it should be?

For processed foods or foods that should be eaten in moderation, try to stick to your size guide and eat the amount of your palm size. For instance, a piece of chocolate cake, a brownie, a cookie, or a muffin should all equal the size of your palm. If the food item comes bigger, cut your appropriate portion and only eat your designated amount. For chocolate bars or candy estimate the size of your thumb. This is like a square of a Hershey's Bar, one or two truffles, or a miniature size candy bar. For high calorie salad dressings or cream based sauces stick to the size of your thumb or 1 tablespoon.

Be sure to check the nutritional information on the back of processed food packages. You'd be surprised how many times you think you're only getting one serving when really a package contains more than one. Your calories double or even triple depending on the amount included. Packaged nuts are a good example.

On the way to a concert my girlfriend, Gaia and I bought a sleeve of mixed nuts from the gas station. The package seemed small, and when Gaia looked at the calories listed, she mentioned 190 calories was not bad for a snack we were sharing. I asked her to tell me how many serving sizes it said and she was shocked to read the package contained three and a half servings. All of a sudden our serving of nuts was much smaller than the package! The entire bag was 665 calories, not 190 calories. Be conscious of the way packaged food is marketed and always be sure to read the label to know if the package contains more than one serving. You can bet that most of the time it does!

Strategy 23

Variety and Moderation

Eating correct portion sizes and decreasing calories need not mean decreasing taste, satisfaction or even ease of meal preparation. Strive for variety to help you achieve your goals without compromising taste, convenience, or nutrition.

When moderation is practiced, it's easy to implement variety into your nutrition. There is room for a little bit of everything. The greater the variety of foods you eat, the less boring and more nutritious! Refer to your food list often to try different types of grains or new vegetables. Try not to get into a rut by just eating the usual corn or beans you are used to. When you get bored with your meals, you'll have a greater tendency to go back to old eating habits.

Try and include as many different food types at each meal. Prepare a vegetable, fruit, whole grain, and healthy protein. After having one serving of everything, if you are still physically hungry, add an additional serving of vegetables or whole grains. You can always add to your meal plate. Avoid setting yourself up to overeat by starting with too large of a serving.

As you implement this new way of eating, pay attention to how your body feels as you see physiological changes occur (fat loss). Healthy eating can be easy since nearly each type of whole food category has convenient options. An effective time saver tip is to use pre-cut fruits and vegetables and pre-packaged salads. Buy as much whole food pre-packaged or pre-cut as possible to make things easy. (Some pre-packaged fruits and vegetables come bottled or in air tight bags and can be found in the refrigerated section of grocery stores.)

BodyJoy Tip

Pick whole foods first when selecting the majority of your snacks. Start with vegetables and fruits, then whole grains, legumes, seeds and nuts.

Healthy Foods List

Vegetables

- Asparagus
- Beets
- Bell Peppers
- Bok choy
- Broccoli
- Brussels sprouts
- Cabbage
- Carrots
- Celery
- Collard Greens
- Corn
- Cucumbers
- Kale
- Leeks
- Lettuce and other greens
- Onions
- Potatoes
- Squash
- Spinach
- Tomatoes
- Any frozen packages
- Frozen Stir-Fry packages
- 100% vegetable juices

Fruits

- Apples
- Apricots
- Bananas
- Blueberries
- Cantaloupe
- Cranberries
- Grapefruits
- Grapes
- Guavas
- Honeydew
- Kiwi
- Lemons
- Limes
- Mangoes
- Nectarines
- Oranges
- Peaches
- Pears
- Pineapple
- Plums
- Raspberries
- Strawberries
- Watermelon
- Any dried fruits (without added sugar)
- Any frozen packs
- Canned fruit in natural or light juices
- 100% fruit juices

Whole Grains

- Grains
  o Rice
  o Oatmeal
  o Wheat
  o Rye
  o Barley
  o Buckwheat
  o Bulgur
  o Flaxseed
  o Millet
  o Amaranth
  o Quinoa
  o Teff
  o Kamut
  o Spelt
- Breads, Bread sticks, Bagels, Rolls, Muffins, Waffles
  o 100% Multi-grain
  o 100% Whole Wheat
  o 100% Whole-grain

- o 100% Sprouted grain
- o Rye
- o Oat
- o Bran
- Tortillas (100% whole wheat or non-fried corn)
- Pizza crust (100% whole grain, wheat)
- Rice (brown, Basmati, Wild, Pilaf)
- 100% Whole grain granola bars
- Oatmeal (whole)
- Couscous (whole grain)
- Cereal (whole wheat, mixed grains)
- Pasta (whole grain)
- Bread and pancake mixes (whole wheat flour)
- Crackers (whole grain, cracked wheat)

Lentils

- Mixed Beans
- Black beans
- Edema me
- Kidney beans
- Lima beans
- White beans
- Pinto beans
- Peas
- Snap peas
- Navy beans

Dairy

- Low-fat milk, yogurt, cheese
- Light and no sugar added yogurt
- Soy dairy products (milk, cheese, yogurts)

Healthy Proteins (look for natural)

- All raw seeds and nuts
- Eggs (omega3 fortified when possible)
- All fresh fish
- Air-tight packaged fish
- Lean, Low fat and fat free choices of meats
  - o Tenderloin
  - o Top round
  - o Sirloin
  - o Turkey breast
  - o Chicken breast
- Meatless bacon
- Meatless sausage links and patties
- Vegetarian burger patties
- Vegetarian hotdogs

Spices and Other Staples

- Any fresh spices
- Basil
- Bay leaves
- Cinnamon
- Cumin
- Curry powder
- Dill
- Vegetable bouillon
- Garlic
- Ginger
- Paprika
- Pepper
- Tomato Paste
- Low-Sodium Broth
- Stewed or Diced Tomatoes
- Low-Sodium Taco Seasoning

Condiments

- Stevia (replacing sugar)
- Canola Oil
- Extra Virgin/Cold Pressed Olive Oil
- No Additive Fruit Preserves
- Agave Nectar
- Honey
- Marinades
- Fat-Free or Soy Mayonnaise
- Mustard
- Natural Butter-Flavored Sprinkles
- Mrs. Dash
- Soy Butter
- Pickled Relish
- Salsa
- Vinegar: Balsamic, Herbed, Fruited, Rice
- Pasta Sauce

Healthier Treats and On-The Go Food Choices (in their correct amounts, of course!)

- Organic dark chocolate (Rapunzel or Endangered Species Brand Bars)
- Air-popped popcorn
- Foodshouldtastegood® whole grain crackers
- Whole grain granola bars
- Stretch Island Fruit Leathers
- Cracked wheat crackers
- Jay Robb Protein Powder
- Amy's Kitchen Frozen Food Meals
- Just Veggies® dried vegetables

- ProBar Whole Foods Meal Replacement Bar
- Odwalla Whole Foods Meal Replacement Bars
- Cliff Nectar Bars (snack bar)
- Organic or raw trail mix

Strategy 24

Make Healthy Eating Easier

A number of my clients have come to realize planning, patience, and persistence are equal payoffs. When it comes to losing fat, a little planning goes a long way. Make things easier on yourself by recognizing you need to spend a little time planning your meals, grocery shopping, and preparing food. Preparation is vital to your success.

Preparation to eating healthy does not have to be time consuming and difficult. It can be done with a modest amount of planning. This strategy provides easy, convenient options to make healthy eating possible if you are on the go, in a restaurant, or at home. To build your daily meals and weekly menus, start with the basics. Refer to this section often for new ideas or as a reminder when you are ready for more variety. My website, *www.mindybuxton.com* also provides ideas and recipes to make healthy eating easy and convenient.

Choose Whole Foods First

Choose whole foods as often as possible. For instance, choose whole wheat rather than white bread, an orange rather than orange juice, baked potato rather than French fries. Think the 80/20 rule. Eighty percent of the time, eat whole foods and twenty percent of the time anything goes. Keep in mind if the food is not in its simple form it counts as a processed food. (French fries are not potatoes and chicken nuggets are not healthy proteins!)

Try getting in all of your servings of fruits, vegetables, and whole grains before eating other food choices. When you do opt for processed foods, stick to your serving size!

Pay Attention to Portions

The amount of food you eat has more to do with if you can lose inches and body fat than any other factor. Keep servings or portion sizes to the size of your palm and the size of your thumb.

Variety

There is no perfect food. As good as broccoli is for you it doesn't have all the nutrients necessary. All foods contain specific nutrients. Eat a variety of foods.

Moderation

You may eat chocolate, candy or chips in moderation; it can fit into your healthy meal planning. Simply balance out your refined sugars with healthy food choices the majority of the time. Concentrate on fruits and vegetables and save sweets for limited treats.

Use Healthy Oils and Spices in Place of High Calorie Sauces or High Sodium Salt

Use healthy types of oils when preparing foods. These include canola oil, olive oil, flax seed oil, corn oil, nut oils, and soy oil. Sometimes you can get away with using olive oil cooking spray in place of oil. Rather than covering your food with salt and unhealthy, high-calorie shortening or margarine, try switching to natural butter or soy butter and using herbs and seasonings for flavor. Use salsa, low sodium taco seasoning, and other healthier toppings to enhance the flavor of your dishes. Regardless of what you use, remember the appropriate serving amounts!

BodyJoy Tip

Frequently take note of what's missing from the fridge or pantry. Having a stock of healthy whole food staples prevents relying on calorie-packed takeout.

Grocery Shopping Tips

- Healthy eating starts with your grocery shopping. Shopping for a simple, whole foods based diet can be less expensive than staples for a traditional American or Western diet.
- Go grocery shopping! If YOU do the shopping, you can control what is available in your house.
- Make time to go grocery shopping when you're not hungry.
- Make a grocery list and stick to it once you're in the store. This will help you cut down on impulse buying.
- Your grocery list should be 80% whole foods and 20% whatever else you like.
- Spend less time in the grocery store by shopping the perimeters (outer isles) where you find most whole foods.
- Buy items such as fruits or vegetables pre-cut, or ready to use. (Think eating and cooking convenience—make them available with the least amount of work!)
- Stick to small amounts/bags of processed treats, even bite sized or miniature when available. Don't buy economy sized processed food treats. (Use Costco and Sam's Club for your fruits and veggies!) Look at the value of not having the amount of tempting treats in your house, not the volume of how much you get for what you pay.
- Set aside one day each week to do your food preparation. (Sort foods into baggies, make soup or bulk salad, cut melons, etc.) Make sure it gets done even if you personally don't do it.

Restaurant Tips

- Try eating out less. Your calories will automatically decrease!
- Choose lower calorie dishes as starters, like vegetables or a salad with dressing on the side.
- Avoid filling up on chips or bread before your meal.

- Take one serving of chips or bread, then have the server remove the rest from you table if your willpower is low.
- Try sharing an entrée.
- Avoid feeling like you have to finish everything on your plate. Take leftovers home for another meal.
- Resist the temptation to super size or upgrade portions of fast foods. Save the .25 cents and the extra 360 calories.
- Avoid unlimited refills on sodas. Switch to water (or better yet, start with water). It isn't worth the extra calories!
- Ask questions about how foods are prepared.
- Ask for substitutes or changes to your order.
- Pass on fried foods and go for steamed or grilled options.
- Make selections from the "healthy choice" section of the menu.
- Ask for more veggies and half the cheese on pizzas.

In the Work Place Tips

- Have a scheduled lunchtime plan and don't work while eating.
- Brown bag or take your lunch to work two or three days each week.
- Take advantage of the office fridge and microwave for storing and preparing healthy snacks.
- Stock a desk drawer with snacks high in fiber, and other nutrients—for example, peanut butter, whole foods meal replacement bars, almonds, dried fruit, apples, oranges, and whole-wheat crackers.
- When you find yourself "lunchless", run to the grocery store rather than a fast food establishment. Select tuna, deli-fresh meats, vegetables, fruits, whole grain crackers or wraps as ideas.

Home Environment Tips

- Make an effort to keep your house or your environment as "safe" as possible by keeping tempting foods that should be eaten sparingly out of sight. Keep them in a cabinet or a drawer that is not used as often as your pantry.
- Store food only in your kitchen, not your bedroom, car, etc.
- Once you get home from grocery shopping, wash and separate produce and/or snack foods into serving size baggies or containers. Make them as easy to grab on the go as processed foods.

- Try not to leave your house for the day without some whole foods snacks such as fruit, vegetables, nuts, or seeds.
- Make your own trail mix out of dried fruits, nuts, and seeds.
- Have a bowl of fresh fruit on your counter.
- Replace your candy dishes with nuts or a healthy trail mix, or remove them altogether.
- Have a batch of healthy vegetable soup made up to use as "tie-you-over-foods" or meals when you are too hungry or tired to cook.
- Plan meals the old-fashioned way: one week's worth at a time. On weekends, buy the groceries you need for at least 4 dinners. Having ingredients in the house means you won't have to resort to high fat takeout.
- Cook once—eat twice. Make enough to have leftovers for sandwiches or fajitas the next day and even the day after that.
- Involve your family in meal planning. If everyone takes more responsibility for meals, they may be more likely to eat them. Assign each family member one night a week to prepare—or at least plan—all or part of a dinner.
- Post the meals you've planned. That way, someone else in the family may be able to get dinner started if you're running late.
- Watch the types of snacks you keep on hand. Fruits and vegetables are preferable to high-sugar soft drinks, potato chips, and muffins.
- Stock up on foods rich in iron, calcium, and fiber, the "problem" nutrients that women and children often lack. Buy calcium-fortified orange juice instead of soda.
- Serve high-fiber cereals for breakfast instead of white toast or high sugar cereals.
- Acknowledge those foods you have a problem with and learn how to manage them in moderation.
- Replace high calorie sauces with flavorful seasonings and spices.
- Serve food dished out on each individual's plate instead of putting serving bowls on the table.

Miscellaneous Tips

- Don't skip breakfast. Breakfast eaters tend to eat less calories and higher fiber amounts than non-breakfast eaters.

- Plan your meals. Haphazard eating usually means choosing foods based on their availability and how they taste—not paying attention to the nutrients they contain.
- Take a multi-vitamin.
- Don't let yourself get too hungry to where you eat haphazardly.
- On days you have little activity, eat less calories. You don't need them unless you are burning them!
- Never let a "splurge" ruin your entire healthy eating plan. Enjoy your short break and get back on track for the next meal.
- Drink plenty of water.
- When you go for a snack ask yourself, "Have I had enough fruits or vegetables today?"
- Experiment with new foods. There's a world of vegetables you've probably never even tried.
- Eat your foods at a slow leisurely pace.
- Rework favorite recipes into healthier versions.
- If you have a favorite "treat" food, keep it in an out of site place, and eat it in small amounts—if you love it, don't give it up, just eat it better!
- Watch your consumption of juices, sodas and alcohol—beverages contain calories.
- Choose monounsaturated fats—avocados, olives, olive oil, hazelnuts, almonds, and peanuts—over trans-fatty acids and saturated fats.
- Consider topping cereals and salads with ground flaxseed for the omega-3 fatty acids, which are essential to good health and help protect against heart disease.
- Use lettuce leaves in place of bread or tortillas on occasion.
- Go vegetarian at least once a week.

Adding Flair and Flavor to Dishes

Consider topping salads or entrees with the following additions:

- Squeeze juice of lemons, limes, or oranges over salads and foods
- Add chunks of canned or fresh fruit such as oranges, pears, apples
- Add slivered almonds or walnut pieces
- Add sunflower seeds and pumpkin seeds
- Add diced tofu

- Add chopped dried fruits such as dried apples, pears, raisins, cherries, or figs
- Add canned beans such as kidney (white or red), cannelloni beans, black beans, etc.
- Use shredded red cabbage
- Use grated carrot

Using Vegetable and Fruits even more by:

- Including tomato and lettuce to sandwiches and veggie or turkey burgers
- Adding chopped apple or pickle to tuna or tuna salads
- Adding mushrooms, chopped tomato, broccoli, diced carrots, diced zucchini, or raisins to rice, bulgur, or other grains
- Serving raw vegetable sticks such as celery, carrots, snow peas, zucchini or cucumbers with salsa instead of chips or high calorie dips
- Opting for fruit as a side to sandwiches rather than fries
- Substituting meat in spaghetti sauce with diced tomatoes, grated carrots, chopped zucchini, or mushrooms
- Adding green, red, or yellow peppers, broccoli florets, sliced carrots, cucumbers, cubed squash, and diced celery to pasta dishes or salads

Use Spices for Flavor

Spices can add wonderful flavor to foods rather than using heavy, high calorie sauces. Rather than covering food in sauces, first go to your spice cabinet for added flavor. Remember that whole foods have an array of different flavors and textures. Try enjoying the flavor and taste of foods naturally. You may be surprised with how little flavor additions you really need.

Time Saver Snack Ideas

- Light string cheese
- Handful of nuts or almonds
- Baggies of raw vegetables (snap peas, celery, carrots, radishes, peppers, etc.)
- Grape tomatoes

- Lunchmeat rolls
- Hard-boiled eggs
- Piece of fruit
- Baggies/Tupperware of cut fruit
- Whole grain granola bars
- Whole Foods meal replacement bar
- Protein bars
- Protein shakes
- Whole wheat/grain/cracked wheat crackers

List 10 Tips you will incorporate today to improve your nutrition.

1. _____

2. _____

3. _____

4. _____

5. _____

6. _____

7. _____

8. _____

9. _____

10. _____

Strategy 25

Finding Your Best Body and Experiencing BodyJoy

Now that you understand that diets will never lead to permanent fat loss and improved health, how do you implement this new healthy meal plan? First things first, make your commitment to abandon dieting and begin eating healthy today. Clean out your fridge and pantry and get rid of the food products that do not promote health and fat loss.

Place the tempting items that lead you away from healthy choices in an obscure place and keep them out of site on a regular basis. Make a grocery list of the supplies and foods you need to begin making more whole-foods based, healthy, high nutrient meals. Begin separating your food into serving size baggies and make sure healthy snack choices are available to you and your family.

Map out a few lunch and dinner menus so you are not stuck last minute without any ideas of what to prepare. Collect healthy recipes that are quick and easy. When you go grocery shopping, add the ingredients to your list so that you'll be sure to get what you need to utilize them.

Begin scheduling your workout time among your daily events. Rearrange what you need to so exercise and activity may occur on a regular basis.

Changing your eating habits and creating a healthier lifestyle is not just about what you take out or stop doing. It's all about what you add in to your routine. It's about doing a little more physical activity, eating more vegetables, and eating appropriate portion sizes.

Know you have the power to make positive changes in your life and remember these few tips for success:

> Choose whole foods first.
>
> Eat breakfast every day.
>
> Exercise regularly, nearly every single day.

Your body's health and fitness is something you will deal with for the rest of your life. What choice will you make? Will you choose to put forth an effort to make time for health and fitness or will you live with the consequences of poor health and an over-fat body? (By the way, the second is definitely more expensive, less fulfilling, and causes you great inconvenience as you age!) With this information, you have the power to overcome the dieting epidemic and never have to participate in the unending cycle of losing body fat and regaining it again. You can experience body joy.

Just remember your fitness and health is ever changing. Be real with yourself and acknowledge that you'll experience highs and lows, successes and plateaus along your journey to your best body. Progress and setbacks cycle as nutrition and activity levels change. Approach it with the attitude of progression, not perfection. As long as you are moving in a positive direction you will succeed in achieving your goals. Embrace these changes that will bring you joy, positive results, and self-respect.

You don't have to do it alone! One of the most important aspects of my program is that you have continual support as you are working on your goals. Throughout these pages I have referred to my website. Log on to *www.mindybuxton.com* and find the support you need. You have access to a weekly newsletter, online personal training support, education and information, and tips from people going through the same process you are. I know how necessary a support system is and I would love you to be part of mine!

Just remember, we can't change how the body is wired. It's a natural urge for the body to hoard calories. It's designed to protect itself against starvation. That's why controllable factors such as exercise and portions are so important. You want to lose body fat and inches? All you need is to make a few changes. These changes will help you feel better, look better and function better as well. These changes will help you create a better experience and lead you to body joy!

As I said before, preparation, patience, and persistence will equal payoffs. You now have the knowledge to incorporate this successful method into your life. Start today and continue to change your body, health and quality of life. As Ralf Waldo Emerson said, *"The First Wealth is Health,"* and you are the only person who can make you healthy and/or wealthy—it's all in how you look at it! Good luck and good health.

Six-week Do-It-Yourself BodyJoy Makeover

Week 1

Identify which type of eater you are.
Weigh In. Get measurements and body fat assessed.
Commit to not weighing yourself until week 6.
Decide if you need exercise equipment or gym access and arrange to purchase or order it.
Write Down 3 Self-Talk Quotes
Make copies of the Daily Log and begin tracking information.
Create a weekly exercise plan. Include 4 days of exercise.
Assess environment. Move or get rid of tempting items/foods.
Go shopping for whole foods.

Week 2

Make 7 copies of the Daily Log and track information.

Create exercise week and include 4 days of exercise.

Assess food section of daily log to see how many fruits and vegetables you are getting.

Try a new vegetable this week.

List ideas to combat behavioral eating types.

Add 3 new self-talk quotes to your list.

Review and/or fill out Body Image section.

Watch *Super Size Me: A Film of Epic Proportions* (Released 9/28/04)

Set goal by filling out goal sheet

Week 3

Make 7 copies of the Daily Log and track information.

Create exercise week. Include 5 days of exercise. Add one interval cardio workout.

Assess food section of Daily Log and see how many fruits and vegetables you are getting.

Add 3 new self-talk quotes.

Read Positive Perceptions and Self-Talk Chapter.

Read Miscellaneous Healthy Tips, choose three to work on.

Week 4

Make 7 copies of the Daily Log and track information.

Create exercise week. Include 5 days of exercise. Have 3 strength training workouts this week.

Assess food section of Daily Log and see how many fruits and vegetables you are getting.

Read "Making Healthy Eating Easy Restaurant and Grocery Tips." Pick 3 to work on.

Add 3 new self-talk quotes. Daily, practice Mental Imagery exercise from "You are an Athlete Section."

Assess how you feel. Are your workouts getting easier? Do you feel more energetic? What are the benefits you are receiving from the past 3 weeks?

Week 5

Make 7 copies of the Daily Log and track information.

Create exercise week. Include 5 days of exercise. Keep 3 strength training workouts this week and add one interval cardio workout to the mix.

Assess food section of Daily Log and see how many fruits and vegetables you are getting.

Read "Rest and Recovery" chapter.

Add 3 new self-talk quotes.

Acknowledge the hard work and effort you are making. Give yourself credit for committing to your goals and doing what it takes to see results.

Week 6

Make 7 copies of the Daily Log and track information.

Create exercise week. Include 5 days of exercise. Keep 3 strength training workouts this week, one interval cardio workout and try something new for your other workout.

Assess food section of Daily Log and see how many fruits and vegetables you are getting.

Add 3 new self-talk quotes.

Acknowledge the hard work and effort you are making. Give yourself credit for committing to your goals and doing what it takes to see results.

At the end of Week 6, make an appointment to weigh in, measure and have your fat percent assessed. Assess your results and keep what worked for you and make changes to what didn't. If you need to set new goals, do it or continue working on your first goal. Acknowledge the changes you've made since week one. Compliment yourself for sticking to 6 weeks! Enjoy your successes and think of what you can do in the next 6 weeks ahead.

Daily Activity Log   *Date*_____

Hours of Sleep   Happiness Level
_____   *Low Moderate High*
Quality of Sleep   Motivation Level
Poor Good Excellent   *Low Moderate High*
Energy Level Cravings
Low Moderate High   *Low Moderate High*
Work Stress Level   Daily Activity
Low Moderate High   *Low Moderate High*
Personal Stress Level (relationships, finances, communication, etc.)
Low Moderate High

Exercise Information

Activity	Category (Strength, Cardio, etc.)	Duration	Intensity

Log Notes from day:

Daily Food Log

*Date*_____

Time	Food	Amount	I Feel...

Strategy 26

Sample Meal Ideas

Breakfasts

- Veggie Omelet with piece of fruit
- Plain oatmeal with almonds or raisins on top with a piece of fruit
- Bowl of high fiber cereal with fruit
- Fruit smoothie with hardboiled egg
- Bowl of fresh fruit with a handful of nuts
- Breakfast burritos with fruit salad

Lunches

- Grilled Chicken Salad with piece of fruit or cup of vegetable soup
- Broth based soup with side salad or some fruit or ½ ProBar
- ProBar or other whole foods meal replacement bar with piece of fruit

Dinners

- Tenderloin or turkey breast
- Barley or basmati rice

- Steamed asparagus or edema me
- Tossed salad with oil and vinegar dressing
- Apple slices

o Wheat tortilla soft tacos with tomatoes, salsa, black beans, soy burger fill
o Steamed mixed vegetables
o Side of fruit
o Salad

- Miso Soup
- Steamed edema me
- Stir fry vegetables over basmati or pilaf rice

o Fajitas
o Fresh fruit salad
o Corn on the cob
o Carrot and celery sticks to dip in salsa

- Whole wheat pasta with kidney beans, mushrooms, and olives
- Tomato Pasta Sauce
- Salad with fresh vegetables covered in limejuice
- Mandarin orange slices

o Tostata on non-fried corn tortilla
o Salmon/Halibut/Tuna Tacos

If you don't have time for a cooked breakfast in the morning, have one for dinner! Try omelets or breakfast burrito meals in the evening!

Snacks

- String cheese and handful of nuts
- Rolled turkey slice with raw vegetables
- Cut vegetables
- Piece of dark chocolate
- Celery stick with peanut butter or hummus
- Bowl of vegetable soup
- ½ whole foods meal bar like ProBar
- Air popped pop corn

BodyJoy Helpful Tips or Recommendations

These tips are in no specific order, just recommendations that have helped me on my journey to BodyJoy.

- Use salsa as a salad dressing
- If you are going to eat processed foods/sugar, keep it to morning and lunch time.
- For an easy last minute dinner, toss some of your already made fresh salad into a frying pan and make a stir fry out of it. You can add a protein to it or keep it vegetarian.
- Find a way to exercise almost daily.
- Train for some type of event or race to make your workouts more purposeful and fun.
- A workout partner is a must! The accountability and support is priceless.
- Jay Robb protein powder is my favorite in terms of taste and purity.
- One piece of an organic dark chocolate truffle can curb any sugar craving.
- Make your water bottle your best friend and never go anywhere without it.
- Know that you will have unhealthy eating moments.
- Know you can overcome those unhealthy moments, forgive yourself, get over it and move on to clean eating as quickly as possible.
- Try the *Healthy Chocolate Chip Oatmeal Banana Cookies* from my Boot Camp Food Manual as an alternative to granola bars.

Additional Recommended Resources

Harris, Barbara, *Shape your Life*, Weider Publications, Inc., Carlsbad, CA, 2003

Robins, John, *The Food Revolution*

Moss, Stephen, *The Power of One*

Egoscue, Pete, *Pain Free*

Spurlock, Morgan, *Super Size Me, A Film of Epic Portions DVD*, release date 9/28/04

Tuttle, Carol, *Remembering Wholeness*

Chek, Paul, *How to Live, Eat, and Be Healthy*

Buxton, Mindy, *The BodyGym Instructor Training Manual*

Vegetarian Cooking for Dummies

The New Mayo Clinic Cookbook

Buxton, Mindy, *Boot Camp Food Manual*

Edwards Brothers Malloy
Thorofare, NJ USA
August 23, 2012